# Aids to Anaesthesia
## 2. Clinical Practice

D0525581

# Aids to Anaesthesia
## 2. Clinical Practice

## M. J. Harrison
MB BS, FFARCS

Senior Lecturer and Consultant Anaesthetist, Nottingham Health Authority and the University of Nottingham, Nottingham

## T. E. J. Healy
BSc, MD, FFARCS, DA

Professor and Head, Department of Anaesthesia, University of Manchester; Honorary Consultant Anaesthetist, Manchester Teaching Hospitals, Manchester, UK; formerly Reader in Anaesthesia and Honorary Consultant Anaesthetist, University of Nottingham, Nottingham, UK; Examiner, Primary Fellowship Examination of the Faculty of Anaesthetists, Royal College of Surgeons of England

## J. A. Thornton
MD, FFARCS, DA

Professor and Head, Department of Anaesthesia, The Chinese University of Hong Kong, Hong Kong; formerly Professor and Head, Department of Anaesthesia, University of Sheffield, Sheffield, UK; formerly Examiner, Primary and Final Fellowship Examinations of the Faculty of Anaesthetists, Royal College of Surgeons of England

CHURCHILL LIVINGSTONE
EDINBURGH LONDON MELBOURNE AND NEW YORK 1984

CHURCHILL LIVINGSTONE
Medical Division of Longman Group Limited

Distributed in the United States of America by
Churchill Livingstone Inc., 1560 Broadway, New
York, N.Y. 10036, and by associated companies,
branches and representatives throughout the
world.

© Longman Group Limited 1984

All rights reserved. No part of this publication may
be reproduced, stored in a retrieval system, or
transmitted in any form or by any means,
electronic, mechanical, photocopying, recording
or otherwise, without the prior permission of the
publishers (Churchill Livingstone, Robert
Stevenson House, 1-3 Baxter's Place, Leith Walk,
Edinburgh EH1 3AF).

First published 1984

ISBN 0 443 02879 6

British Library Cataloguing in Publication Data
Harrison, M. J.
   Aids to anaesthesia.
   2: Clinical practice
   1. Anesthesia
   I. Title    II. Healy, T. E. J.    III. Thornton, J. A.
   617'.96    RD81

Library of Congress Cataloging in Publication Data
Harrison, M. J.
   Aids to Anaesthesia.
   Includes index.
   CONTENTS: pt. 1. The basic sciences.—pt. 2. Clinical practice
   1. Anesthesia—Handbooks, manuals, etc. I. Healy,
T. E. J. (Thomas Edward John) II. Thornton, J. A.
(John Andrew) III. Title. [DNLM: 1. Anesthesiology—
Handbooks. WO 200 H318a]
RD82.2.H37    617'.96    83-7202

Printed in Singapore by Selector Printing Co (Pte) Ltd

# Preface

This book is intended to aid candidates in the final preparation for postgraduate examinations in the clinical practice of anaesthesia.

The application of physiological and pharmacological concepts to medical problems in clinical anaesthesia is dealt with on a functional basis; the pathophysiological/pathopharmacological 'defect' is identified and the measures intended to minimise the hazard due to the disturbance are presented.

A more conventional approach is used in the description of techniques used in the practice of anaesthesia, pain relief and intensive care.

We do not presume to have included all the knowledge required for the examinations, other texts fulfil this function. This book is an *aide-mémoire*.

The authors would like to acknowledge the care taken by Mr Geoffrey Lyth of the Department of Audiovisual Aids in the Medical School, University of Nottingham, who prepared the illustrations, and by Mrs J. A. Shore for much of the typing. Thanks are also due to Dr Ian Fletcher for his help with the index.

Nottingham, Manchester
and Hong Kong, 1984

M. J. H.
T. E. J. H.
J. A. T.

*Dedicated, in gratitude, to our mothers*

# Contents

# 1. Principles of general anaesthesia

The classical 'triad' of anaesthesia, 1) hypnosis, 2) analgesia and 3) suppression of reflexes (autonomic and neuromuscular transmission), may be extended to include a fourth component of anaesthetic practice—the maintenance of gaseous exchange. The use of drugs, with a single primary effect such as hypnosis, analgesia or neuromuscular blockade, may be combined in low doses (balanced anaesthesia) to allow the minumum effective dose of each to be used, thereby avoiding the need for a relatively larger dose of a single drug.

## HYPNOSIS

*Hypnotic agents* induce sleep by non-specific depression of the central nervous system. Hypnotic agents usually have no analgesic action. Respiratory and cardiovascular depression may occur, particularly if used in association with other drugs which have a central depressant effect. Hangover effect may occur as may tolerance, psychological dependence and enzyme induction. The last mentioned may lead to the rapid metabolism of other medication including oral anticoagulants, corticosteroids, digoxin, oestrogens and androgens.

### Hypnotics used to induce general anaesthesia

*Barbiturates* (thiopentone, methohexitone, hexobarbitone)
Water-soluble salts of barbituric acid (Fig. 1.1) are produced by substitution of aryl or alkyl radicals for hydrogen or oxygen atoms.

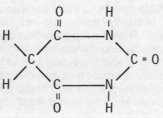

**Fig 1.1** Barbituric acid

They are water-soluble salts. Depression of synaptic transmission in the reticular activating system leads to sleep. Sensory pathways are not depressed and therefore there is no analgesic effect—indeed the pain threshold may be reduced.

The EEG initially shows barbiturate activation (fast activity) but with loss of consciousness slow waves (delta rhythm), similar to those seen in physiological sleep, occur.

Barbiturates used to induce general anaesthesia (hexobarbitone, methohexitone and thiopentone) have a high lipid-water solubility coefficient and therefore the onset of effect is rapid (10 s), but because they bind to plasma proteins they are rapidly distributed to other tissues, e.g. muscle and fat, and therefore have a brief duration of action (thiopentone 5–10 min) in spite of a relatively slow metabolism (15% of thiopentone dose metabolised per hour). Methohexitone has a more rapid metabolic clearance (1–2 hours). Those barbiturates that are used to induce anaesthesia are almost completely metabolised. Excretion is increased in the presence of alkaline urine.

Thiopentone dissolves to form an alkaline solution which is irritant to tissues—extravasation may lead to tissue sloughing. Intra-arterial injection may cause intense vasoconstriction with thrombosis, leading to gangrene of the limb extremity (finger tips). Treatment includes direct intra-arterial injection of vasodilating agents such as 2% procaine, papaverine or 5 ml tolazoline (1% solution) and blockade of the sympathetic nerves (stellate ganglion block). Hexobarbitone and methohexitone are less irritant than thiopentone. The use of these drugs may be associated with laryngospasm, hiccough and abnormal muscle movements. The latter being more common with methohexitone.

### Benzodiazepines (diazepam, lorazepam)
Benzodiazepines have many actions in common, although the degree to which a particular action predominates varies from drug to drug. They have anxiolytic, anticonvulsant and muscle relaxant (central effect) properties but no significant analgesic effect. Intramuscular absorption is poor in spite of good oral absorption. Highly protein bound, many of these drugs have a prolonged plasma half-life ($T\frac{1}{2}$) and are metabolised to active metabolites which also have a prolonged $T\frac{1}{2}$. Enterohepatic circulation and hepatic storage may lead to reappearance of the effects of the drugs after apparent recovery. Side-effects include sedation, muscle weakness, amnesia, confusion, allergic phenomena and slight depression of the respiratory system. Their action may be potentiated by other central depressants. Benzodiazepines are used as hypnotics, anxiolytics, premedicants, anticonvulsants and to control athetoid movements in spasticity. Variation in response to a given dose makes diazepam and lorazepam unsatisfactory for use as induction agents. Benzodiazepines are also noted for their amnesic effect.

*Phencyclidine derivatives* (ketamine)
Ketamine is an induction agent which may be administered orally,
i.m., i.v. or p.r. It has analgesic, cataleptic and hypnotic actions.
During recovery from anaesthesia vivid dreaming and irrational
behaviour may occur. Unconsciousness follows within 30 s of
intravenous injection and lasts for about 5 min. Recovery follows
redistribution with subsequent metabolism to active metabolites. In
spite of having, like other anaesthetic agents, a generalised
depressant effect, tachycardia with a rise in blood pressure usually
follows an i.v. injection of ketamine. This paradoxical action is at
least in part due to noradrenaline re-uptake blockade. It may
therefore have a use in the presence of bronchospasm, but should
be avoided in hypertensive patients.
    Its anticholinergic action may augment the effect of
neuromuscular ganglion blocking agents.
    Diplopia and nystagmus may also occur as may tonic and clonic
muscle movements.

*Eugenol derivatives* (propanidid)
Propanidid has rapid onset with short duration of effect after i.v.
injection. Propanidid is insoluble in water but is soluble in
cremophor EL. There is rapid hydrolysis ($T\frac{1}{2}$ = 5 min). Breathing is
initially stimulated but depression follows. Tachycardia occurs and
though CVS depression is uncommon it may occur precipitously,
often associated with anaphylactoid-type reactions. It may cause
local irritation to blood vessels and postoperative nausea. The
effect of suxamethonium is prolonged.

*Steroids* (Althesin)
Alphaxalone is formulated with alphadalone (Althesin) for i.v.
injection. It is insoluble in water but soluble in cremophor EL. Rapid
metabolism limits the effect to about 10 min. There is no
discomfort on injection. The respiratory and cardiovascular
systems are normally stable, though acute hypersensitivity
reactions may lead to cardiovascular collapse and severe
bronchospasm. Postoperative nausea may also occur. Althesin has
no corticosteroid properties.

*Carboxylated imidazole* (etomidate)
Etomidate has a rapid onset of action after i.v. injection, with rapid
recovery, but creates little change in the respiratory or
cardiovascular systems. However it may produce involuntary
movement and local pain during intravenous injection.

## ANALGESIA

Drugs which relieve pain are known as *analgesics* and these may be considered to be of two types:
a) The antipyretic or anti-inflammatory analgesics, which are primarily used for pain of musculoskeletal origin and act through a peripheral mechanism
b) Narcotic or morphine-like analgesics, which are primarily used for pain of visceral origin and for pre-, post- and intra-operative pain; they act through a central mechanism

### Antipyretic/anti-inflammatory analgesics
Acetylsalicylic acid is a convenient source of salicylate, an effective analgesic with antipyretic and anti-inflammatory actions. These effects may depend on the inhibition of prostaglandin $E_2$ synthesis, although it may also have a central action. Plasma concentration rises quickly (gastric absorption) and maximum plasma concentration is achieved within two hours. Acetylsalicylic acid is hydrolysed in the gastric mucosa and in the plasma to salicylate. Approximately 60% of plasma salicylate is bound to protein and is rapidly distributed throughout the body. It is important to reduce the dose of other drugs used simultaneously which are also protein bound, e.g. warfarin, as these may be displaced from their protein binding sites by salicylate. Salicylates increase the bleeding time by decreasing platelet adhesiveness and by reducing plasma prothrombin levels. Renal excretion of salicylate is encouraged by an alkaline urine, and conversely, in an acid urine, reduced ionization of salicylate leads to reduced excretion.

Salicylate stimulates breathing by a direct central action and by increasing oxygen utilization and carbon dioxide production. There is also uncoupling of phosphorylating mechanisms. In salicylate poisoning there may be a metabolic acidosis, a respiratory alkalosis and occasionally there may be a rise in $P_a\text{co}_2$ with a fall in pH. Overdose may lead to headache, dizziness, tinnitus, thirst, nausea and skin eruptions.

### Narcotic analgesics
Morphine and drugs with a similar action are known as narcotic analgesics. The effects and potencies of such drugs are usually compared to morphine as the standard. Use of drugs of this type may lead to physical dependence.

*Natural alkaloids*
Only 4 of 20 opiate alkaloids in the seed capsule of the opium poppy (*Papaver somniferum*) have a clinical use. These are morphine, codeine, noscapine (narcotine) and papaverine.

Morphine
Central effects include analgesia, euphoria, sedation and
depression of the cough reflex, respiratory centre and vasomotor
centre. Nausea, vomiting and miosis occur. Oliguria is associated
with the release of antidiuretic hormone. Peripheral effects include
reduced gastro-intestinal tone, spasm of the biliary tract and
contraction of the sphincter of Oddi. Histamine release may lead to
bronchospasm. Labour is retarded. Morphine is concentrated in the
lungs, liver, kidneys, spleen and skeletal muscle. Hepatic
conjugation is followed by excretion primarily in the urine and less
in bile. A single dose of morphine is largely excreted within 24 h.

Methylmorphine (codeine)
It is less potent than morphine, its metabolic product, and is used
for cough suppression. It may cause constipation.

Papaveretum
Papaveretum contains the water soluble alkaloids of opium. The
analgesic effect depends on morphine (50% of the mixture).

*Semi-synthetic narcotic drugs*

Diacetylmorphine
Diamorphine is more lipid soluble than morphine and is better
absorbed orally. It is converted to morphine, is more potent and
sedative than morphine, but causes less respiratory depression.

Dihydrocodeine
It is more potent than codeine but has very little respiratory or
cardiovascular depression.

*Synthetic compounds*

Pethidine
Pethidine has a shorter duration of action than morphine but is less
likely to produce spasm of smooth muscle. Nausea, vomiting and
sedation occur.

Fentanyl, alfentanil, phenoperidine
These agents are used to supplement $N_2O$ analgesia. Their potency
exceeds morphine by factors of 80, 20 and 10, respectively.
Alfentanil has the shortest onset and duration, phenoperidine the
longest duration. These drugs are related to pethidine, respiratory
depression and muscle rigidity may occur. Haemodynamic stability
and rapid recovery are notable. Mono-oxidase inhibitors should be
avoided.

Benzmorphan derivatives (pentazocine)
Pentazocine is an opiate like analgesic with antagonistic properties

and may therefore precipitate the withdrawal syndrome in opiate addicts. Hallucinations may follow its use. It may be administered intravenously, intramuscularly, subcutaneously or orally.

Thebaine derivative (buprenorphine)
A very potent analgesic with equal agonist and antagonist properties. In addition to analgesia buprenorphine produces sedation, respiratory depression and miosis. However, effective analgesia may occur in association with negligible respiratory depression. There is a very low incidence of vomiting, and dysphoria and hallucinatory effects have not been reported. It may be administered i.v., i.m., s.c. and sublingually.

A single dose provides prolonged pain relief, thereby reducing the need for repeat injections.

## NEUROMUSCULAR BLOCKADE

Muscle relaxation in the context of anaesthesia may be interpreted as reduced muscle tone. The tone in a muscle is adjusted by proprioceptive responses and voluntary control. Muscle tissue is depressed by general anaesthetic agents and therefore deep anaesthesia is associated with a reduction in the muscle tone and in the force of artificially-induced contraction. Interference in the motor nerve pathway will reduce the muscle contraction response. Traffic through the motor pathway may be reduced by the use of centrally-acting muscle relaxants such as diazepam, although it is more usual to use neuromuscular blocking agents. Diazepam has no direct effect on the neuromuscular junction. Motor impulse transmission can also be intercepted in the nerve fibres within the vertebral canal by by the use of local anaesthetic agents injected into either the subarachnoid or the epidural space.

Neuromuscular transmission is mediated by a chemical transmitter (acetylcholine) released from the nerve ending. Acetylcholine is synthesised in the nerve ending where it is stored in vesicles; when it is released by an action potential in the nerve it diffuses to the motor end-plate on the muscle surface. The motor end-plate is a highly specialised area of the post-synaptic membrane. The attachment of acetylcholine to the specialised receptors leads to a change in the membrane permeability to sodium ions and depolarisation occurs. The depolarisation process is propagated across the muscle fibre and muscle contraction results. Acetylcholine is rapidly hydrolysed by an esterase and repolarisation of the membrane takes place.

The drugs used during general anaesthesia which act directly at the neuromuscular junction are of two types:

### Depolarising agents
Depolarising agents produce depolarisation of the end-plate membrane and then prevent repolarisation, thereby maintaining

blockade of neuromuscular transmission. Recovery follows drug hydrolysis by plasma cholinesterase. Effective drugs include suxamethonium, suxethonium and decamethonium. Their effects may be potentiated by agents which alter neuromuscular transmission, or which inhibit plasma cholinesterases such as trimetaphan, phenactropinium, hexafluorenium and tetrahydroaminacrine (tacrine), neostigmine, physostigmine and ecothiopate iodide eye drops.

Unwanted prolongation of the effect may be associated with the use of propanidid, aprotinin, cyclophosphamide, quinidine, procainamide, procaine and amethocaine.

a) Suxamethonium
b) Suxethonium

These two drugs have a similar effect which is short-lived and terminated by drug hydrolysis. Suxamethonium may be injected as a bolus dose or administered as a 1% infusion to maintain relaxation. The use of suxamethonium may be associated with severe postoperative muscle pains. The incidence of muscle pain may be reduced by the i.v. injection of 3 mg of d-tubocurarine before the injection of suxamethonium.

The action of suxamethonium may be prolonged if cholinesterase activity is impaired. Reduced plasma cholinesterase levels are associated with severe liver disease, chronic anaemia and cardiac failure, bronchial neoplasia, starvation, exposure to organophosphorous compounds including ecothiopate iodide, radiotherapy and treatment with immunosuppressive and anti-cancer agents.

A low level of plasma cholinesterase activity may be associated with an atypical cholinesterase. This condition occurs in about 1 in 3000 patients and is genetically determined by a pair of non-dominant allelomorphic autosomal genes. The atypical cholinesterase is able to hydrolyse acetylcholine at the concentration normally present in the plasma, but its ability to hydrolyse drugs at therapeutic concentrations may be markedly reduced. The activity of the atypical enzyme is dibucaine (cinchocaine) resistant, whereas the activity of the common enzyme is inhibited by dibucaine. This fact provides a basis for identifying the presence or absence of an atypical gene.

Malignant hyperpyrexia may follow the use of suxamethonium.

**Non-depolarising agents**
Non-depolarising relaxants are bound to the postsynaptic membrane but do not excite a change in membrane sodium permeability, so that depolarisation does not occur. However, access by acetylcholine to the receptors is reduced. An equilibrium exists between acetylcholine and the muscle-relaxant drug such

that an increase in the available acetylcholine following administration of an anticholinesterase (e.g. neostigmine) alters the equilibrium and the block is reduced. Effective drugs include d-tubocurarine, gallamine, alcuronium, pancuronium fazadinium and atracurium. The neuromuscular blocking effect may be potentiated by other agents which are anti-cholinergic (anti-nicotinic), which include drugs with a ganglion-blocking action such as trimetaphan, phenactropinium and ketamine. Agents with a calcium ion antagonist action may directly influence the muscle contractile elements and in addition reduce acetylcholine release and thereby potentiate the non-depolarising relaxants. Agents which act in this way include the aminoglycoside antibiotics, disopyramide, verapamil, nifedipine. The effect of muscle relaxants may also be modified by lithium salts and by the intravenous injection of local anaesthetic agents.

a) D-tubocurarine
Mild hypotension may result from a combination of ganglion blockade and histamine release. This drug should therefore be used with care when combined with drugs which lower blood pressure, and caution must be exercised in the presence of phaeochromocytoma or a history of bronchial asthma. The effect is reduced by alkalosis and prolonged by acidosis.

b) Gallamine
A marked tachycardia follows injection of this drug. This agent should not be used during obstetric anaesthesia because it freely enters the fetal circulation. It is predominantly excreted by the kidneys and therefore should be avoided in the presence of renal failure. Effect is prolonged by alkalosis and reduced by acidosis.

c) Alcuronium
Similar in action to d-tubocurarine but less hypotension and less histamine release are produced.

d) Pancuronium
More rapid in onset than d-tubocurarine. Does not lead to histamine release or hypotension. Tachycardia and a rise in blood pressure may occur, as a result of noradrenaline reuptake blockade.

d) Pancuronium
Similar action to d-tubocurarine with histamine release and ganglioplegic action. Use is frequently associated with hypotension and tachycardia.

f) Atracurium
A highly selective non-depolarising muscle-relaxant that is degraded spontaneously by a non-enzymatic decomposition

process (Hofmann elimination) to inactive products. Its breakdown is not dependent on metabolism, liver or kidneys.

## INHALATIONAL ANAESTHETIC AGENTS

Some inhalational agents at low concentrations possess hypnotic properties but at higher concentrations produce analgesia and muscle relaxation. Others in low concentrations produce analgesia and little hypnosis, trichloroethylene and methoxyflurane for example. Muscle relaxation, however, may be achieved only at levels which alter the respiratory and cardiovascular reflexes. Potency is expressed in terms of the MAC value, i.e. the minimum alveolar concentration of the agent, at equilibrium, required to prevent 50% of patients moving during a 'standard' skin incision at normal atmospheric pressure. The oil/gas partition coefficient bears a close relation to the MAC value.

### Nitrous oxide
A gas, neither flammable nor explosive, stored as a liquid under pressure at room temperature. The blood/gas solubility coefficient of 0.41 explains the rapid induction, but on the other hand its low potency is reflected in the high MAC value (MAC 101). Nitrous oxide is a good analgesic at inspired concentrations of 50–70% but has no effect on skeletal, cardiac or uterine muscle.

During recovery, nitrous oxide diffusion into the alveoli may reduce alveolar oxygen tension ($P_AO_2$) and lead to hypoxia (diffusion hypoxia—Fink effect).

### Diethyl ether
A volatile liquid (boiling point 35°C) flammable in air. Induction and recovery are slow (blood/gas solubility coefficient 12.1), but its potency is high (MAC 1.9). Diethyl ether is irritant to the airway but nonetheless produces bronchodilatation. Raised sympathetic tone masks the depressant effect on the heart. Respiratory depression occurs at high dose.

### Trichloroethylene
A volatile liquid with a boiling point of 87°C, neither flammable nor explosive at concentrations used clinically. Induction and recovery are slow (blood/gas solubility 9.15), but potency is high (MAC 0.16). Recovery is further slowed by metabolism to tricholoroethanol and trichloroacetic acid. Tachypnoea may occur, as also may ventricular dysrhythmias, particularly if high concentrations are used, or in the presence of hypercarbia and increased adrenaline levels. Adrenaline should not be injected in patients breathing trichloroethylene. Trichloroethylene reacts with soda lime to produce dichloroethylene and phosgene, a cranial nerve poison,

and should therefore be avoided if a rebreathing circuit with soda lime is used.

## Halothane

A volatile liquid with a boiling point of 50.2°C, neither flammable nor explosive. Induction and recovery are rapid (blood/gas solubility 2.3 and potency is high (MAC 0.77). However, tachypneoa may lead to reduced alveolar ventilation, and as the inhaled concentration is increased, myocardial depression may result in hypotension. The fall in cardiac output is related to a reduced stroke volume. Ventricular dysrhythmias may occur in the presence of increased adrenaline levels and therefore adrenaline should not be injected during halothane administration, except under cover of beta adrenergic blockade. Halothane depresses skeletal, cardiac and uterine muscle. There is evidence that repeated halothane anaesthetics over a short period may sensitise the patient to halothane and lead to hepatic changes.

## Enflurane

A volatile non-flammable liquid with a boiling point of 56.6°C. Induction and recovery are fast (blood/gas solubility coefficient 1.9) and potency is high (MAC 1.68 in 70% nitrous oxide). It produces a dose-related depression of tidal volume, respiratory rate and myocardial contractility. Sensitisation of the myocardium to adrenaline is less than with halothane. Enflurane depresses skeletal, cardiac and uterine muscle and potentiates muscle relaxants. Metabolic products include inorganic fluoride, but the concentrations of this do not reach nephrotoxic levels. An abnormal EEG, a seizure pattern, may occur at high concentrations. Enflurane does not appear to affect the normal liver.

## Methoxyflurane

This poorly-volatile liquid (boiling point 104°C) is non-inflammable in air provided the concentration remains below 4% at a temperature of 75°C. Induction and recovery times are prolonged (blood/gas solubility 13.0) but the potency is high (MAC 0.16). This agent depresses ventilation with increasing dose and may produce hypotension. On the other hand, it is a good analgesic and muscle-relaxant. Nephrotoxicity may occur and cause high output renal failure. Two MAC hours has been suggested as the upper dose limit.

## PREOPERATIVE CONSIDERATIONS

Many factors influence preoperative assessment, preparation and premedication.

50% of patients presenting for surgery have a pre-existing medical condition and a drug history can be obtained from 60%.

The medical assessment and preparation of patients and possible drug interactions are dealt with in Chapter 2. Patients normally take nothing by mouth from midnight prior to anaesthesia; for afternoon surgery a light early breakfast (06.00 hrs) is sometimes allowed. This regimen can put certain patients at risk, particularly the newborn, and intravenous fluid and nutrients should be given.

Urgent procedures in the unstarved patient present a dilemma; the stomach of the patient at great risk should be emptied. The passage of a nasogastric tube may induce vomiting, although unless it is of a very large size it will not facilitate the emptying of the stomach directly. Apomorphine, an emetic, has been used, but is also unpleasant. Metoclopramide is an agent that may speed the emptying of the stomach and has some use.

Premedicant drugs are used for the control of secretions, for the alleviation of anxiety and to produce a foundation on which to construct the anaesthetic.

Atropine, hyoscine and glycopyrrolate are all used as anti-siallogogues. Their desirability in premedication is debatable. A dry mouth is uncomfortable and more likely to be traumatised. Atropine has been associated with a fall in oxygen saturation and hyoscine can produce confusion in the elderly.

Anxiolytic agents, although on superficial assessment they may appear ideal, have also been shown to produce a significant fall in arterial oxygen tension and should therefore not be given to those patients with limited cardiorespiratory reserve. Similarly opiate premedication may be associated with respiratory depression. A pre-operative visit by the anaesthetist is efficacious and without adverse side-effects.

## ADMINISTRATION OF ANAESTHESIA

Induction of anaesthesia is generally produced by intravenous injection of one of the induction agents mentioned. Care must be taken to avoid intra-arterial injection, or extravascular injection into the median nerve, if the injection is to be made in the antecubital fossa. The risk of intra-arterial injection, though much reduced, is still present if a vein on the back of the hand is used.

Inhalational inductions employ either air, or nitrous oxide and oxygen as carrier agents. To be a useful induction agent, a volatile liquid anaesthetic agent requires a high vapour pressure at room temperature, a low blood/gas solubility coefficient and a low MAC value (e.g. halothane, 2.3 and 0.77, respectively). The tidal air alone may be used to carry the vapour, either in an open system using a Schimmelbusch mask, or in a draw-over apparatus, such as the EMO (Epstein McIntosh Oxford) vaporiser.

Drugs which produce general anaesthesia usually also produce respiratory and cardiovascular depression. Patients with limited respiratory or cardiovascular reserve are therefore particularly at risk.

If an inhalational induction is used the pulmonary ventilation and the cardiac output will infuence the rate at which the anaesthetic agent is taken up, and hence the time to induce anaesthesia. The rate of induction is directly related to the alveolar minute volume and inversely related to the cardiac output. The use of an intravenous induction agent may obviate the ventilatory and circulatory factors, but on the other hand may cause cardiovascular and respiratory depression, thereby not only affecting the subsequent introduction of inhalational agents, but in some circumstances could threaten the patient's survival.

The basic but essential concepts upon which the administration of every anaesthetic must be constructed are depicted in Figs 1.2 and 1.3. These may be summarised as follows.

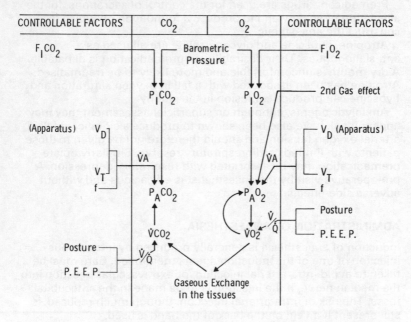

Fig 1.2  Factors influencing gaseous exchange in the respiratory system

## 1. Protection of alveolar ventilation and oxygenation

a) Control of the patency of the airway
b) Maintain adequate tidal volume ($V_T$) and frequency (f) with limitation of the apparatus dead space ($V_D$) or provision for carbon dioxide absorption
c) Provision of an effective oxygen concentration ($F_IO_2$) in the gas and anaesthetic mixture

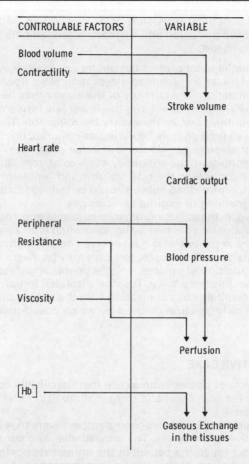

**Fig 1.3** Factors influencing gaseous exchange in the cardiovascular system

## 2. Protection of oxygen delivery to the tissues

a) Correct deficiency in haemoglobin by transfusion. Desaturation and anaemia can result in a dangerous fall in the quantity of oxygen available to the tissues. This can only be compensated for by increasing the cardiac output through an increase in cardiac work.

b) Maintenance/correction of blood volume. Perfusion can only be maintained if venous return, hence cardiac output, is maintained.

c) Assess adequacy of cardiac output and where necessary support with inotropic and chronotropic agents. Maintain heart rate > 40 and < 160 per minute.

d) Control of peripheral resistance. Vasoconstriction leads to reduced tissue perfusion and a greater afterload puts extra strain on the heart.

The anaesthetist must protect the patency of the airway. Obstruction of the airway leads to a cessation of air flow and hence of alveolar ventilation. The patency of the airway may be ensured by the simple expedient of holding the lower jaw forward (not by closing the mouth), or when necessary by intubation. The fractional content of gases inhaled may be varied as required, but breathing is essential for alveolar ventilation and in the presence of respiratory depression, the adequacy of alveolar ventilation must be ensured by controlling the tidal volume and ventilatory frequency. Apparatus dead space should be reduced to a minimum to reduce rebreathing of expired alveolar gas.

'Balanced anaesthesia' using muscle-relaxants and small doses of hypnotic/analgesic agents may be associated with awareness during surgery. A patient who has received no premedication and only nitrous oxide with a muscle relaxant may be aware during surgery. The addition of opiates, volatile agents and dissociative agents reduces this possibility. Tunstall's isolated forearm technique to facilitate communication with the patient during surgery is the only practical method by which consciousness can be detected.

## POSTOPERATIVE CARE

The two aspects of postoperative care that specifically concern anaesthetists are pain relief and oxygenation. Pain relief is dealt with in Chapter 4.

Drugs administered both pre- and peroperatively may contribute to postoperative hypoxaemia. The anaesthetist, and surgeon, should have access to the patient in the immediate postoperative period and a high nurse/patient ratio is mandatory, 1:4 or higher. $P_aO_2$ may fall by 3 kPa (22 mmHg) as a result of a residual large right to left shunt in the pulmonary circulation.

Hypoxaemia is greater in the elderly, and greater after thoracic and upper abdominal surgery. A reduction in functional residual capacity and the loss of the pulmonary vasoconstrictor response to hypoxia caused by anaesthetic agents are thought to be the main causes.

Medium concentration oxygen masks should be used routinely for those at risk, but oxygen therapy alone should not be used to compensate for respiratory depression due to any cause. Respiratory stimulants such as doxapram may have a place but it will not overcome inadequate reversal of non-depolarising muscle-relaxants and should be used with great care in patients with hypertension or tachycardia.

Posture was thought to be an important factor in postoperative hypoxaemia, i.e. sitting or lying, but recent work has cast doubt on this. Good pain relief certainly helps the patient but may not improve oxygenation; airway obstruction is probably the commonest cause of severe acute hypoxaemia and should always be avoided. Shivering and increased muscle tone can lead to hypoxaemia.

Maintenance of cardiac output by correct fluid management and the avoidance of myocardial depressants also minimises hypoxaemia.

## ANAESTHESIA IN THE NEONATE

Apart from the generally more fragile structure, there is a marked difference in the anatomy of the airway, making intubation more difficult. The larynx is positioned rather more anteriorly than in the adult and higher, under the posterior aspect of the tongue. Laryngoscopy is achieved best by using a straight bladed laryngoscope, the blade being placed behind the V-shaped epiglottis. The epiglottis is flattened by the blade, allowing the glottic opening to be seen. Laryngoscopy is hindered further by the relatively large neonatal head which causes anterior neck flexion, leading to soft tissue obstructing the view of the glottis. This may be overcome by placing a small pillow behind the shoulders, the head being supported at a lower level, thereby extending the neck over the pillow. It is important to secure the endotracheal tube in three planes so as to reduce movement, and therefore laryngeal trauma, to a minimum. For this reason nasal intubation is frequently used, particularly if prolonged ventilation is anticipated. A cuffed endotracheal tube, which would reduce the diameter of the airway, increasing the resistance to airflow, is not used. For positive pressure ventilation an airtight fit is achieved between the walls of the larynx and the tube in the region of the cricoid cartilage, the narrowest part of the neonatal larynx.

The apparatus dead space must be reduced to a minimum. Even a few millilitres of apparatus dead space, which may be no hazard in an adult, may markedly reduce the alveolar ventilation when the tidal volume is itself only 20 ml, the physiological dead space 5 ml and the minute ventilation in the order of 400 ml (2.5 kg neonate).

### Heat-loss

The surface area of a neonate is much greater relative to its body weight than the adult surface area. The relatively large surface area together with the higher skin temperature may lead to excessive heat loss. Loss of heat combined with an immature temperature-regulating centre may in a cold environment lead to a fall in temperature. As body temperature falls, hyperkalaemia, hyperglycaemia and acidosis result. It is essential therefore to monitor the body temperature, using an oesophageal or rectal thermometer, and to reduce heat-loss during anaesthesia and surgery of the neonate by the use of a warmed operating theatre, constant body temperature blankets, cotton wool insulation and aluminium foil. Heated blankets must not exceed 42°C. The neutral temperature of the environment is between 34° and 35°C for neonates compared with 29°C for adults.

## Monitoring
Laboratory assessment of plasma sodium, potassium, chlorides, glucose, proteins and blood urea may be valuable in monitoring electrolyte imbalance, dehydration and the response to treatment. The blood urea may rise markedly in postmature babies and may vary considerably with pyrexia and marginal dehydration. The neonatal kidney may not be able to cope with a sodium load and therefore it is important in planning the intravenous fluid regime to avoid administering a sodium overload during and after surgery. A 5% sugar solution may be all that is required. It is important to remember that when prolonged gastric secretion or vomiting have occurred sodium and chloride replacement may be necessary. The neonate also excretes potassium less efficiently than the adult, and indeed the plasma concentration of potassium may be considerably raised following surgery. The calcium requirement is generally met by the milk diet, but in the presence of severe diarrhoea calcium may be supplemented intravenously if shown to be necessary. The magnesium requirement is not usually a matter for concern, though in the presence of faecal fistula or an ileostomy magnesium replacement may be required.

## Fluid replacement
The total body water and extra-cellular water constitute higher proportions of the total body weight in the neonate than in the adult. Insensible loss generally amounts to 100 ml per day and this volume in addition to the volume of urine produced should be replaced. However, when the neonate is nursed in an incubator with an atmospheric humidity approaching 100%, insensible fluid loss may be halved. Urine output increases from approximately 20 ml on the second day of life to 150 ml on the seventh day. In general terms, on the first postoperative day during the first week of life fluid replacement may be calculated on the basis of 40 ml.kg$^{-1}$. In older babies the fluid replacement volume is calculated on the basis of 165 ml.kg$^{-1}$. The volume given may need to be reduced during the postoperative period if urine production is reduced.

The neonate's initial blood volume is dependent upon transfusion from the placenta. The haemoglobin value may be 20 g.dl$^{-1}$; however this is reduced progressively by haemolysis. The fall in value is most rapid during the first 2 weeks of life and at 3 months the value may have fallen to 10 g.dl$^{-1}$ blood.

## Anaesthesia

Preoperative assessment should include weight, temperature, respiratory and cardiovascular status and the presence of twitching (hypocalcaemia, hypoglycamia, hypoxia). Atropine 0.15 mg is normally given as premedication with vitamin K if less than 3 days old.

General anaesthesia is not generally required for intubation of the neonate but in older babies either an inhalation or intravenous induction may be used. The thoracic cage is very pliable and this may lead to a marked reduction in the pulmonary functional residual capacity, and therefore hypoxia with cyanosis may occur very rapidly when ventilation is interrupted. This effect is further augmented by the relatively higher pulmonary vascular resistance and an initial right to left shunt. Spontaneous ventilation in the neonate depends largely on the diaphragm. Rib excursion is limited by the horizontal position at rest and by the distortion resulting from diaphragmatic contraction. Ventilation is normally controlled using a muscle-relaxant and is monitored using an oesophageal or praecordial stethoscope. The most commonly used breathing system is the T-piece (Ayre 1937). For spontaneous ventilation a gas flow of 3x $\dot{V}$ prevents $CO_2$ retention. The Rees modification (reservoir bag with through flow) facilitates controlled ventilation. Higher flows are used to ensure no $CO_2$ retention (3–41.min$^{-1}$).

Effective oxygenation, with any ventilatory interruption reduced to a minimum, remains a primary duty of the anaesthetist. The maintenance of blood volume is similarly of major importance, and blood loss must be measured, by weighing of swabs or by a colorimetric method.

## Surgery

There are several conditions that need surgical intervention in the first two months of life.

1) Pyloric stenosis
2) Exomphalos
3) Gastroschisis
4) Tracheo-oesophageal fistula
5) Congenital diaphragmatic hernia
6) Congenital cystic disease of lung
7) Developmental abnormalities of spine and cranium
8) Hydrocephalus (insertion of pressure relief valve)

The detailed management of these conditions cannot be covered adequately in a book of this nature, but the fundamental concepts of managing the newborn remain the same. Anaesthesia for some of these conditions is covered in Chapter 3.

## ANAESTHESIA IN THE ELDERLY

The two limits of life, i.e. the neonate and the elderly, in some ways reflect each other. The elderly patient is generally more fragile than the younger adult. Fragile skin and blood vessels lead to more rapid bruising and brittle bones are more likely to fracture. Advanced degenerative diseases—cardiac, pulmonary, vascular, cerebrovascular, renal and hepatic—may be present, in addition to frank cardiopulmonary disease, low-grade chronic renal and pulmonary infection, muscle wasting, frequently associated with inanition, and anaemia, making anaesthesia and surgery more hazardous in the elderly and dictating the need for the most careful pre-operative assessment.

A degenerative process reduces the functional reserve of the system affected, and therefore the onset of disease in a system already damaged by a degenerative process is more likely to lead, at an early stage, to frank failure. Hence the elderly with arteriosclerosis are less tolerant of hypoxaemia, particularly in low flow states or if the perfusion pressure is inadequate.

Cardiac failure is common in the elderly and is often associated with coronary artery disease and loss of muscle volume, which follows coronary blood vessel occlusion, with fibrous replacement. Furthermore, arteriosclerosis affecting the aortic valve and aorta may limit the cardiac output. The elderly therefore have an impaired myocardial functional reserve and may not be able to adjust to sudden changes in blood volume, hypo- or hyperthermia, to the negative inotropic effects of drugs such as thiopentone and halothane, to active diseases, including sepsis, or to the increased metabolic demands following surgery. It may therefore be considered valuable to digitalise all elderly patients before surgery. A positive inotropic effect may be expected even in the absence of obvious cardiac failure. All patients with atrial fibrillation should be digitalised.

The elderly lungs are also subject to degenerative changes and to frank disease. Airway closure occurs when the intrapleural pressure (dependent on gravity and the volume of the chest) exceeds the critical closing pressure (dependent on elastic recoil) and thus in the elderly, in whom elastic tissue is lost, airway closure occurs at a higher lung volume. When closing volume exceeds the functional residual capacity, airway closure is then taking place during normal tidal flow.

Closing volume (% of total lung capacity) = 19.4 + 0.5 (age)

At 65 years the closing volume exceeds the FRC when standing, there is therefore inefficient gas mixing and $P_{AO_2}$ falls.

Pulmonary changes in disease usually lead to either increased airway resistance (obstructive) or reduced pulmonary excursion (restrictive) and associated pulmonary vascular disease. Chronic bronchitis and emphysema are the most common presentations. However, the presence of pulmonary fibrosis or neoplasia and associated intrathoracic disease, including a pleural effusion, must be considered. A careful assessment of pulmonary and cardiopulmonary function is vital. Pre-operative pulmonary preparation to improve breathing and reduce infection is essential in all but emergency situations. Blood transfusion, fluid and electrolyte therapy may be required to correct anaemia, dehydration and electrolyte imbalance. Anaesthesia should be instituted and maintained in such a way that further impairment of cardiovascular compensation is reduced to a minimum. Intermittent positive pressure ventilation may be required to ensure adequate oxygenation and the prevention of hypercarbia. Heat loss should also be reduced to a minimum. Confusion is not uncommon in the elderly and may have many causes. However it may be precipitated by sedative or anxiolytic drugs. Hyoscine should be avoided.

Local anaesthetic techniques have been shown to have advantages over general anaesthesia in the elderly—the morbidity and mortality associated with spinal anaesthesia being less for hip surgery than general anaesthesia. It is advisable to avoid the sympathetic blockade associated with higher blocks because of the obtunded vasomotor responses in the elderly. Local anaesthesia spreads higher in the elderly, whether spinal or epidural, and thus volumes of local anaesthetics should be modified accordingly.

Early postoperative mobility is essential.

## ANAESTHESIA IN PREGNANCY

### 1. First trimester
It is wise to avoid the administration of any drug during the early part of pregnancy. However, there is no evidence to suggest that the administration of a general anaesthetic carries a specific teratogenic risk. Association between teratogenesis and anaesthetic agents is not conclusive and generally relates to prolonged exposure, as experienced by operating theatre staff. If a member of staff is planning to become pregnant it is advisable that she avoids the theatre/recovery room/intensive care environment, particularly in the first months of pregnancy.

### 2. First and second trimester
Miscarriage may be associated with general anaesthesia, particularly if intra-abdominal surgery is performed.

### 3. Third trimester
*Supine hypotension*
The uterus may, if the patient lies supine, obstruct the inferior vena

cava and thereby impair venous return. The resultant fall in cardiac output may lead to severe hypotension. The incidence of this eventuality can be reduced by tilting the operating table, and hence the patient, to the left. Supine hypotension only occurs in a minority of patients and these patients are thought to lack collateral vessels bypassing the inferior vena cava. Aortic compression may also add to the reduction in placental perfusion caused by the hypotension.

*Increased acid secretion*
The dangers of gastric acid inhalation (described by Mendelson in 1945) have been well-documented. It is not always possible to plan anaesthesia in pregnancy and patients may therefore have had a recent meal. Furthermore, gastric emptying is slowed and, owing to the distortion of the diaphragm caused by the large uterus, the cardia may be less effective in preventing regurgitation. Regurgitation and inhalation of gastric contents may therefore occur. This likelihood must be reduced. In the first instance the pH of the stomach contents may be raised by oral antacids, sodium citrate (30 ml of 0.3 molar solution) is the present antacid of choice. Direct stomach emptying with a gastro-oesophageal tube is not normally considered necessary, neither is the use of apomorphine, an emetic, but circumstances may dictate that this is necessary, e.g. a recent meal, a known intubation difficulty and urgent surgery all in the same patient.

Atropine is now thought to reduce the tone of the gastro-oesophageal sphincter. Glycopyrollate has been reported to raise the pH of the gastric contents.

Pre-oxygenation before induction of anaesthesia will obviate the need for positive pressure oxygenation, which may encourage gastric emptying by squeezing the stomach between the diaphragm and the other abdominal contents, including the large uterus. Cricoid pressure should be applied to prevent regurgitation into the oropharynx during induction, or induction should be carried out with the patient in the lateral position.

*Fetal gas exchange*
Gas exchange between maternal and fetal blood takes place in the placenta. The umbilical artery blood gas tensions are 16 mmHg (2 kPa) $P_aO_2$ and 46 mmHg (6 kPa) $P_aCO_2$. These values are altered to 29 mmHg (4 kPa) $P_aO_2$ and 42 mmHg (5.5 kPa) $P_aCO_2$ in the umbilical vein as a result of the oxygen and carbon dioxide gradients which exist between the fetal and maternal blood. (*Note*: the umbilical venous blood has been described using arterial symbols because it is analogous to the blood in the pulmonary vein).

The *double Bohr effect* facilitates oxygen transfer to the fetus:
The transfer of fetal carbon dioxide to the maternal circulation moves the maternal oxygen haemoglobin saturation curve to the

right, thereby reducing the affinity of maternal haemoglobin for oxygen which releases oxygen. On the other hand, the rapid transfer of carbon dioxide across the membrane increases the affinity of fetal haemoglobin for oxygen, thereby facilitating the transfer of oxygen across the placental membrane.

A similar mechanism facilitates carbon dioxide transfer to the mother—the double Haldane effect—but is not quite so effective because of low levels of carbonic anhydrase in the fetus.

### Cardiovascular changes during pregnancy

A marked increase in cardiac output (30–40%) may occur in association with a rise in blood volume (50%), salt and water retention, and a fall in the haemoglobin concentration. Retraction of the uterus after delivery may therefore constitute a major fluid overload. The vasoconstricting effect of ergometrine may therefore be contra-indicated and oxytocin preferred.

### Effects of drugs on the uterus and fetus

In general terms overdose of anaesthetic, analgesic and sedative drugs will depress uterine contractions. It is therefore important to use drugs in the minimum effective therapeutic dose. Halothane, enflurane and trichloroethylene can be used safely in low concentrations. Thiopentone is similarly unlikely to effect uterine muscle tone if minimal sleep doses are used. Indeed the effect of thiopentone on the fetus is likely to be of greater importance than its effect on the uterus. Ketamine disobeys the general rule and is reported to increase uterine muscle tone. Narcotic agents, when used in normal therapeutic doses, are unlikely to effect uterine contractions and can be used safely. However, in higher doses, uterine and fetal depression may occur.

Drug transfer to the fetus across the placenta depends on its lipid solubility, its degree of ionisation and its protein-binding properties, as with any other membrane. It also depends on the timing of the injection if the patient is in labour. A drug injected just prior to a contraction may not reach the placenta at all. Detoxification of drugs may occur in the placenta as amine oxidases and esterases are present.

There is evidence that suggests that benzodiazepines are not good for the fetus: diazepam and lorazepam have both been associated with low APGAR scores at birth.

# 2. Problems associated with medical disease processes

There are innumerable diseases, but limited numbers of gross physiological effects. Not all of these effects are of relevance to anaesthesia.

The following is an attempt to catalogue the physiological/pharmacological disturbances of relevance to anaesthesia.

Drug interactions
Acute adverse reactions to drugs
Altered sensitivity to drugs
Upper airway problem
Lower airway problem
Failure of oxygenation (respiratory)
Critical ventilatory ability
High cardiac output
Fixed cardiac output
Low cardiac output
Failure of oxygenation (cardiovascular)
Abnormal vasomotor control
Reduced oxygen carriage
Increased risk of thrombosis
Increased risk from haemolysis
Disorder of haemostasis
Reduced ability to co-operate
Increased risk of cerebral damage
Altered metabolic state
Australia antigen
Increased risk of renal failure
Skeletal problems
Skin and mucous membranes at risk

## INTERACTIONS BETWEEN THERAPEUTIC AGENTS AND AGENTS USED IN ANAESTHESIA

### Antacids

*Sodium bicarbonate*
This antacid, in excess, can cause systemic alkalosis and thus may influence the effects, duration and excretion of other ionised drugs.

## Antibiotics

The following antibiotics have been shown to interfere to various degrees with neuromuscular transmission.

| | | |
|---|---|---|
| Amikacin | Gentamycin | Polymyxin B |
| Bacitracin | Kanamycin | Streptomycin |
| Clindamycin | Lincomycin | Tobramycin |
| Colistin/colymycin | Neomycin | Tetracycline |

## Anticholinesterases

*Ecothiopate iodide eyedrops*
Ecothiopate may interfere with the action of neuromuscular blocking agents which should therefore be used with care.

## Antidepressants

*Tricyclics*
The re-uptake of noradrenaline is inhibited by these drugs. They may cause potentiation of sedatives and sympathomimetic agents, the latter leading to hypertension: adrenaline and noradrenaline are absolutely contra-indicated.

There is evidence that the 'tricyclics' increase the incidence of arrhythmias during halothane anaesthesia for oral surgery.

*Mono-amine oxidase inhibitors*
The inhibition of mono-amine oxidase leads to the accumulation of 5HT, dopamine and noradrenaline within the neurone.

Interactions of note may occur with:

Tricyclic antidepressants
Sympathomimetic amines
Levodopa
Pethidine
Morphine
Pentazocine
Phenazocine
  and other narcotic analgesics

If these agents are to be given, discontinue therapy for at least 3 weeks pre-operatively.

*Lithium*
Sodium imbalance may occur.

Toxic levels can potentiate barbiturates and modify the response to neuromuscular blocking agents.

## Antihypertensives

Some may obtund the normal cardiovascular reflexes and increase the sensitivity to general anaesthetic agents, e.g. hydrallazine, methyldopa, reserpine and guanethidine.

Beta adrenergic receptor blockers have been known to induce a myasthenic syndrome and to unmask myasthenia gravis.

Trimetaphan has been shown to potentiate the neuromuscular blocking action of both non-depolarisers and depolarisers. Nitroglycerine prolongs the effect of pancuronium.

Care should be taken with sympathomimetic agents if the patient is taking debrisoquine or guanethidine.

## Anti-Parkinsonian therapy

### Amantidine
Care with concurrent administration of central nervous system stimulants.

### Levodopa
Levodopa may interact with many agents. However, during normal anaesthesia there should be few problems, although, because beta adrenergic receptors in the heart are stimulated, an increased incidence of arrhythmias under halothane anaesthesia has been noted.

Take care if administering antihypertensives or sympathomimetics.

Patients undergoing general anaesthesia should have therapy stopped the night before operation.

### Methixine
Blood pressure may be unstable as there is the possibility of autonomic lability.

## Beta adrenergic receptor blockers

### Cardio-selective

Practolol
Metoprolol
Atenolol

### Non-selective

Propranolol
Oxprenolol
Labetolol

Heart failure can be precipitated by beta adrenergic receptor blockade and bradycardia may limit the heart's ability to respond to large changes in blood volume and/or peripheral resistance.

Care should be taken with all general anaesthetic agents, but diethyl ether and cyclopropane in particular, as these agents normally provoke sympathetic activity.

### Carbenoxolone
Hypokalaemia may occur, which may alter the actions of other agents, such as digitalis.

### Contraceptive pill
Increased risk of deep vein thrombosis

### Digitalis glycosides
Digitalis intoxication leading to disturbances in cardiac conduction, the intestine and the CNS may be precipitated by electrolyte disorders and drugs.

Hypokalaemia, hypomagnesaemia, hypernatraemia, hypercalcaemia and alkalosis.

Diuretics can cause hypokalaemia, as do carbenoxolone, the contraceptive pill, corticosteroids, reserpine and catecholamines.

### Diuretics

*Potassium-sparing*
A relative hypovolaemia may exist, which may be revealed if a vasodilator agent is administered.

*Non-potassium-sparing*
Hypokalaemia and possible hypovolaemia.

### Endocrine therapy

*Glucocorticoids*
Steroid supplementation may be necessary.

*Mineralocorticoids*
Check electrolyte homeostasis and fluid balance.

*Insulin*
Abnormal potassium levels may alter the actions of other agents and thus the potassium concentration should be checked. This problem associated with insulin normally only occurs if an acute diabetic state is being treated.

*Pitressin*
Check electrolyte homeostasis and fluid balance.

## ACUTE ADVERSE REACTIONS TO DRUGS

### Induction agents
Acute adverse reactions must be differentiated from the effects due to relative overdosage or to an exaggerated response to the drug.

The features of acute adverse reaction to intravenous induction agents are bronchospasm, cardiovascular collapse, oedema of the airway (the life-threatening features), erythema, rashes and urticaria (the common but less devastating features).

*Causes*
1. Release of histamine
2. Activation of C3 complement     } Anaphylactoid
3. Immune mediated mechanism     Anaphylactic
   (An anaphylactic reaction requires previous exposure to the agent)

Reporting of reactions to drugs is very incomplete; therefore it is difficult, with certainty, to assess their incidence. Reactions to Althesin, for example, have been estimated to range from 1 in 9 to 1 in 19.

*Management of the acute major adverse reaction*
1. Administer oxygen, intubation may be necessary and IPPV
2. Set up an intravenous infusion—give fluids if hypotensive
3. I.V. aminophylline or s.c. adrenaline for bronchospasm
4. Hydrocortisone
5. Monitor the ECG

Thiopentone and methohexitone, or any other barbiturate, are absolutely contra-indicated in porphyria, a congenital metabolic abnormality. Their use may result in lower motor neuron paralysis, psychic disturbances or possibly death. Etomidate and althesin are also contra-indicated in porphyria, but ketamine and propanidid are considered safe.

**Neuromuscular blocking drugs**
Histamine can be released by both non-depolarising and depolarising agents. If severe the reaction should be treated as described above for anaphylactoid reactions. Pancuronium should not be used in porphyrics.

The most dramatic and life-threatening reaction to the administration of a muscle-relaxant is that of malignant hyperpyrexia in response to the injection of suxamethonium.

*Malignant hyperpyrexia* (MH)
*Incidence* —approximately 1:200 000 in the UK
            —MH may not be induced on the first exposure to drugs
              known to induce it (44% probability)
            —greater in patients undergoing surgery for hernia,
              squint and spinal deformity
            —most patients are of late childhood/early adult age
*Inherited* —autosomal dominant with variable expression

*Induced by*—all volatile anaesthetic agents
          —suxamethonium
          —psychotropic drugs
          —stress— the unknown factor—the absence of this
                 may be responsible for the 56% probability that MH
                 will not be induced in those known to be
                 susceptible
*Indicators* —muscle spasm
          —inappropriate tachycardia
          —tachypnoea
          —cyanosis
          —oozing—Disseminated intravascular coagulation (DIC)
          —arrhythmias, cardiac arrest

Management
Mortality about 50%
Diagnosis—a temperature rise of $> 1°C$ per 10 minutes
        (exclude other causes of pyrexia—infection, atropine
          overdose, hot environment)
        —muscle spasm (exclude other causes—dystrophia
          myotonica, myotonia congenita)
Discontinue inhalational agents and surgery
Hyperventilate with 100% oxygen
Set up intravenous infusion
   $NaHCO_3$ 100 mmol to combat acidosis
   10% dextrose and 20 $\mu$ soluble insulin—to lower $[K^+]$
Take arterial blood sample for acid/base and electrolyte analysis,
   clotting 'screen' and $[Ca^{++}]$.
Dantrolene, 1 mg. $kg^{-1}$ intravenously—this may need to be
   repeated after 5 min (maximum dose 10 mg.$kg^{-1}$). Dantrolene
   may elevate the potassium level.
Methylprednisolone, dexamethasone, or hydrocortisone in high
   dosage.
Active cooling may be necessary

      —droperidol may aid cooling and reduce muscle spasm
      —ice packs in groins, axillae and around neck
      —cool intravenous fluids
      —cold water sponging and enhanced evaporation with fans
      —peritoneal dialysis with cold fluid may be used

Catheterise the patient—save a sample for myoglobin detection
Mannitol 1 g.$kg^{-1}$ intravenously may protect against cerebral
   oedema and renal failure
Inotropic agents may be required (isoprenaline) to maintain the
   cardiac output
Beta adrenergic receptor blockers may be required to treat
   extrasystoles or tachyarrhythmias

Recovery may be prolonged over several days during which fluid and electrolyte balance must be continuously assessed and adjusted. An osmotic diuresis should be maintained, and potassium supplementation will be required. Further dantrolene may be needed, $1-2$ mg.kg$^{-1}$ four times a day.

The patient and relations should be subsequently be investigated by muscle biopsy.

Anaesthesia for the patient susceptible to MH
1. A vaporiser-free anaesthetic machine
2. Monitoring of ECG, temperature, access for arterial blood analysis
3. Means for cooling should be at hand
4. Safe drugs

| | |
|---|---|
| Diazepam, droperidol | —premedication |
| Thiopentone, althesin, fentanyl | —induction |
| 50% nitrous oxide in oxygen | } —maintenance |
| Pancuronium | |

(Do NOT reverse the neuromuscular blockade with neostigmine and atropine)

Local anaesthetic agents may be used—procaine, tetracaine, lignocaine, bupivacaine and prilocaine are considered safe.

**Inhalational agents**
All inhalational agents have been implicated in the genesis of malignant hyperpyrexia, see above.

Other acute adverse reactions are those associated with the irritancy or acute effects of high doses: laryngeal spasm, coughing, breath-holding, bronchospasm and hiccup to name a few. The usual management is to turn the agent off or reduce the concentration appreciably until the condition is brought under control.

Arrhythmias (p. 42) may occur spontaneously but are more likely in association with hypoxia or hypercarbia. Continual monitoring of cardiac action (ECG or pulse monitor) is preferable to intermittent monitoring (finger on pulse).

Halothane and enflurance are contra-indicated in porphyria.

## RESPIRATORY DISEASE

The problems facing the anaesthetist include varying degrees of ventilatory failure with or without associated cardiovascular decompensation, e.g.:

1. Right ventricular hypertrophy/failure (cor pulmonale)
2. Polycythaemia secondary to chronic hypoxia

**Upper airway problems**

*Causes*

CNS depression

Trauma

Infection    These patients may be in danger of spontaneous obstruction

Tumour

Anatomical variations

Trismus

Scleroderma    These patients may be less likely to obstruct spontaneously but may be associated with problems of per-oral endotracheal intubation

Burns

Arthritis

*General approach to the patient with potential airway obstruction*
Heavy sedation is undesirable as control of the airway may be lost. The integrity of the airway is particularly at risk in the unconscious. The use of a naso-pharyngeal airway should be considered.

Nurse in the lateral position where necessary to facilitate drainage of secretions, or blood, in cases of trauma.

*Problems*
Whether the patient to be anaesthetised is to breathe spontaneously or to be ventilated, security of the airway is essential and thus it is mandatory to assess the situation very carefully.

*Management*
1. Does the patient need endotracheal intubation?
   a) to protect the airway
   b) to facilitate surgery
   c) to allow IPPV
   If not, use another technique.
2. Assess the problem
   Nature and size of lesion
   Severity of functional problem, e.g. can a gas-tight fit be made between face and mask?

   In those with cervical or temporomandibular joint arthritis, ankylosis, or those with an abnormal jaw, a lateral X-ray of mandible and cervical spine (in extension and flexion) should be obtained.
   Carry out indirect laryngoscopy, it may be helpful.
3. Premedication—none or only a light anxiolytic/neurolept premedication
4. Pre-oxygenation. The body oxygen store of an adult male in normal respiratory health breathing air is approximately 1500 ml. This can be increased three-fold by administering 100% oxygen to breathe for 3 minutes, or, if 3 minutes is too

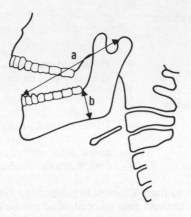

If a/b = <3.6 intubation is
likely to be difficult

**Fig 2.1** Radiological measurements indicating possible difficulty at
endotracheal intubation

  long to wait because of the urgency, then 5 or 6 deep breaths
  of 100% oxygen is almost as good.
 5. Gaseous induction, with or without small i.v. dose of hypnotic
   agent.
   Deepen anaesthesia using halothane or enflurane with the
   patient breathing spontaneously.
 6. Perform direct laryngoscopy when muscular relaxation has
   occurred.
   Visualise the laryngeal aperture.
     Do NOT use neuromuscular blocking agents until the
   endotracheal tube is in position.
 7. Have stylets, bougies, various sizes of tubes and
   bronchoscopes available. Nasal intubation should be
   considered—it may be easier.
 8. If intubation impossible, wake patient up and try intubation
   using local anaesthetic technique.
 9. If still impossible, try trans-cricoid epidural needle technique.
10. Tracheotomy using local anaesthetic.
  Success is enhanced by correct positioning of the patient, by
maintaining oxygenation, by keeping the patient asleep, and by
avoiding damage.

**Lower airway problems**
*Causes*
  Acute/chronic bronchitis
  Bronchospasm (asthma)
  Histamine release

*Problems*
Increased airway resistance may make adequate ventilation difficult

*Chronic bronchitis/emphysema*

Management: Severe respiratory dysfunction makes it advisable to use a regional anaesthetic technique whenever possible. When this is impossible then a controlled ventilation technique should be employed.

Preparation: Lung function tests
$FEV_{1.0}$  $P_aCO_2$  $P_aO_2$
Improve function by physiotherapy, antibiotics, antispasmodics and possibly mucolytics and steroids

Premedication: Avoid opiates that may lead to respiratory depression and/or bronchospasm

Induction: Pain, light anaesthesia, and irritant inhalational agents may induce bronchospasm. Histamine release may also occur.
Intravenous aminophylline (0.4–0.5 g) may be administered. Preoxygenation should be followed by induction with an intravenous hypnotic and suxamethonium. Liberal 'topical' 4% lignocaine should be sprayed over the vocal cords and upper trachea and then endotracheal intubation should be carried out.

Maintenance: Neuromuscular blockade should be produced by gallamine triethiodide or pancuronium and the ventilatory pattern should be that of a prolonged expiratory pause. Minute ventilation should be adjusted to compensate for the increased alveolar dead space. Adequate oxygenation should be ensured by the administration of a 50:50 oxygen: nitrious oxide mixture and the the depth of anaesthesia by 0.5–1.0% halothane.

Reversal: 1. Patients with an $FEV_{1.0}$ <1.0 litre and a $P_aCO_2$ > 5.3 kPa and a $P_aO_2$ < 8 kPa breathing air should be electively ventilated with or without PEEP in the post-operative period.
2. Patients with an $FEV_{1.0}$ <1.0 litre and normal blood gases and no excess bronchial secretions should be 'reversed' with neostigmine, after pre-atropinisation, and graded oxygen therapy should be instituted.

Postoperative care: Conduction nerve block analgesia should be used rather than systemic analgesics.

*Asthma*

| | |
|---|---|
| Assessment: | Frequency of attacks and their control should be evaluated |
| | Drug therapy—steroids—antispasmodics |
| | Respiratory function tests |
| | $FEV_{1.0}$ and the response to therapy |
| | $P_aco_2$   $P_ao_2$ |
| Preparation: | Physiotherapy |
| | Antispasmodics |
| | Inhalational therapy—IPPB with bronchodilators |
| Premedication: | Anxiolytics |
| | Bronchodilator—inhaler |
| | Avoid opiates |
| Induction: | Intravenous aminophylline may be given |
| | Preoxygenation |
| | Methohexitone or diazepam may be considered |
| | Avoid thiopentone, althesin, propanidid |
| | Suxamethonium |
| | 4% lignocaine spray to larynx and trachea |
| Maintenance: | Humidification |
| | IPPV—use pancuronium or gallamine, avoid d-tubocurarine |
| | PEEP may be helpful |
| | Halothane may decrease bronchiolar tone if spasm is present |
| Reversal: | Use neostigmine with care |
| Postoperative care: | Graded oxygen therapy |
| | Conduction nerve block analgesia preferably |

## Failure of oxygenation

*Causes*
V/Q imbalance
   Venous admixture
      Chronic bronchitis/emphysema
      Consolidation/collapse of lung
      Pulmonary oedema
Vascular lung tumour
Hyaline membrane disease
Defects of heart and great vessels (see CVS subsection)

*Problems*
Pulmonary shunting leads to deficient oxygenation of the blood and slowing of the uptake of inhalational agents.

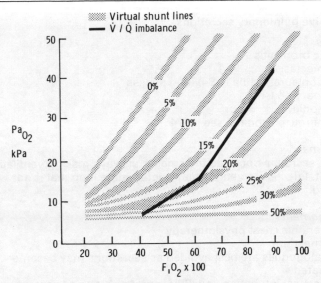

**Fig. 2.2** The relation between $PaO_2$ and $FIO_2$ due to shunts (virtual shunt lines) and $\dot{V}/\dot{Q}$ imbalance (one example shown).

*Management*
Use regional techniques where possible

| | |
|---|---|
| Assessment: | A-a gradient<br>$P_aO_2$ breathing air and oxygen<br>$P_aCO_2$ breathing air and oxygen |
| Preparation: | Aim to optimise pulmonary function with physiotherapy, antibiotics, antispasmodics, mucolytics |
| Premedication: | Avoid respiratory depressants |
| Induction: | Preoxygenation and denitrogenation to enhance the uptake of inhalational agents<br>A LA technique should be used where suitable |
| Maintenance: | Avoid spontaneous ventilation as there is a tendency to underventilation which leads to further atelectasis and greater 'shunting' |
| Reversal: | If endotracheal intubation employed aspirate secretions from tracheo-bronchial tree. If preoperative $FEV_{1.0} <1.0$ litre consider using a respiratory stimulant to maintain adequate alveolar ventilation (i.v. doxapram has been shown to be effective) |
| Postoperative care: | Physiotherapy to the chest and graded oxygen therapy<br>Avoid opiates if possible |

**Excessive pulmonary secretions**

*Causes*
Chronic bronchitis
Bronchiectasis
Bronchopleural fistula (p 94)/lung abcess
Pulmonary oedema
Pneumonia
(Cholinergic poisoning) see p 174

*Problems*
Excess secretions occlude the smaller airways making ventilation difficult. Infected secretions may contaminate lung that is not infected.

*Management*
Pre-operative chest physiotherapy
Treat infection
Anti-sialogogues are best avoided as secretions may become inspissated
Endotracheal intubation and IPPV is preferable to a spontaneous ventilation technique (except for a broncho-pleural fistula, see below)
Tracheal aspiration should be carried out as frequently as required
In unilateral disease endobronchial tubes are used to prevent flooding of the unaffected lung with purulent material or excess secretions.
Endobronchial tubes, see p 190

*Postoperative care*
Physiotherapy to the chest
It may be considered necessary to leave an endotracheal tube in situ, to facilitate the aspiration or clearance of secretions

**Critical ventilatory ability**

*Inadequate spontaneous ventilation*

*Causes*
CNS depression
Disease processes of the spinal cord (Guillain-Barré syndrome).
poliomyelitis
Peripheral neuropathy
Neuro-muscular disease
   myasthenia gravis
   myopathies
Restricted movement of the chest wall
   Crush injury of the chest
   Obesity

Acute lung disease—fulminating pneumonia
Chronic lung disease
Upper respiratory tract obstruction
Diaphragmatic paralysis or immobility
Each of these entities require specific therapy but the functional problem of incipient respiratory failure needs a common approach if surgery is required.

*Problems*
Incipient respiratory failure (failure of oxygenation and/or failure of carbon dioxide excretion) can only be aggravated by anaesthesia and the decision to undertake surgery must be combined with a positive attitude to respiratory support during and after surgery.

*Assessment*
Clinical history and examination
Arterial blood gas measurement
Pulmonary function tests (with exercise tolerance tests if possible)

*Management*
1. Elective ventilation
2. If ventilation is likely to be prolonged—tracheotomy
3. Chest physiotherapy

**Inadequate ventilation with positive pressure ventilation**

*Causes*
Massive leak
    Bronchopleural fistula
    Tracheo-oesophageal fistula (TOF)

*Problems*
Both bronchopleural fistula and tracheo-oesophageal fistula are associated with pulmonary infection, the purulent material in the pleural space soiling the tracheobronchial tree in the former, and food or saliva in the latter. The larger the fistula the greater the soiling and also the greater the air leak should IPPV be instituted. On occasions the leak is so great that ventilation of the good lung is minimal.

*Assessment*
Bronchoscopy may indicate the site and the size of the fistula—but bronchoscopy itself is a hazardous procedure and should be carried out with the patient breathing spontaneously.

*General approach*
1. NEVER paralyse the patient before it is established that positive pressure ventilation can be effectively performed

2. Isolation of fistula by use of appropriate endobronchial tube during spontaneous respiration
3. Testing of isolation of leak by applying positive pressure to airway and assessing leak into
   a) under water seal drain or
   b) into stomach
4. If isolation of leak is complete than IPPV can be instituted

If inflation of the oesophagus via a TOF cannot be avoided then spontaneous respiration should be allowed until surgical access facilities ligation of the fistula.

When ventilating patients with bronchopleural fistula of a diffuse type, i.e. a raw lung surface, then ventilation may be achieved by using a conventional single lumen tube, the ventilator settings should be such that there is a very short inspiratory phase. This ensures optimal distribution of gas throughout the lungs.

## CARDIOVASCULAR DISEASE

Cardiovascular diseases may have effects that involve all other systems and thus the problems with which the anaesthetist is presented are diverse, e.g.:
1. Renal failure associated with hypertension
2. Intestinal stasis due to mesenteric embolisation
3. Cerebral ischaemia due to atheroma
4. Liver dysfunction due to right heart failure/venous congestion

Cardiac output is determined by a combination of stroke volume and heart rate. Blood volume, vascular capacity, venous return and myocardial contractility are some of the many other factors.

### High cardiac output

*Causes*
Tachycardia < 160 b.p.m. (pyrexia, anxiety, exercise, carbon dioxide retention)
Thyrotoxicosis

*Problems*
Slow induction of anaesthesia when using volatile agents
Possibility of high output cardiac failure (Heart failure is the inability to maintain an adequate cardiac output in situation where other cardiovascular variables are normal or where the other variables are so disturbed that the physiological limits on cardiac contraction are exceeded)

*Assessment*
Clinical history and examination
Central venous pressure
Skin temperature

*Preparation*
Specific therapy should be started in an attempt to return the
cardiac output to normal
Agents likely to exacerbate the situation should be avoided, such as
atropine

## Fixed cardiac output

*Causes*
Obstructive valvular heart disease
Fixed heart rate
Constrictive pericarditis
Cardiac tamponade

*Problems*
The general problem is that of the inability to withstand
haemodynamic changes, i.e. the toleration of changes in blood
volume and peripheral resistance is low.
For example:

*Aortic stenosis*
Hypotension should be avoided as myocardial ischaemia increases
thus impairing an already precarious situation.

*Aortic incompetence*
Hypertension should be avoided as this increases the
intraventricular pressure and thus reduces myocardial perfusion.

*Mitral stenosis*
A tachycardia is hazardous as ventricular filling is reduced and the
cardiac output falls.

*Mitral incompetence*
Hypertension and bradycardia lead to an increase in regurgitation
and thus a fall a cardiac output.

*Assessment*
Clinical history and examination
Chest X-ray (heart size, signs of left ventricular failure)
ECG
Specific investigations as necessary
  Phonocardiography
  Cardiac catheterisation

1. Pre-operative preparation should be such that the patient is in
   the optimal state of surgery
2. Sedative premedication is used to minimise the adrenergic
   response to anxiety

3. Preoxygenation should precede induction of anaesthesia
4. The use of intravenous induction agents should take into account the altered circulation time so that the correct dose is administered at the correct speed which in this situation should be very closely monitored
5. Maintenance of general anaesthesia—$N_2O/O_2$/neuromuscular blockade with or without an analgesic + IPPV
6. ECG monitoring during the whole procedure

AVOID
   Hypovolaemia
   Sudden vasodilation
   Chronotropic agents (care with neostigmine and atropine, the use of glycopyrrolate preferable)
   Myocardial depressants such as halothane
   Specific therapy for patients with valvular heart disease should include the use of prophylactic antibiotics to protect against sub-acute bacterial endocarditis.

## Low cardiac output
1. Inadequate contractility
2. Inadequate preload
3. Excessive afterload
4. Inefficient heart rate—< 40 or > 160 b.p.m.

### 1. Inadequate contractility

Causes
Ischaemic heart disease
Cardiomyopathy
Decompensated valvular heart disease

Problems
Arrhythmias
Low output cardiac failure
   Ischaemic heart disease—stable angina, ST segment and T-wave changes have been found to be of minimal importance in determining cardiac risk. A myocardial infarct within 6 months and rhythm disorders, however, are considered high risk factors.
   One third of patients operated on within 3 months of an infarct reinfarct, and half of these die.
   During anaesthesia the heart rate: blood pressure product should be kept below 16000 (HR × BP, 80 × 120 = 9600); this is said to minimise cardiac work; hypotension however is undesirable, as coronary perfusion is compromised.
   Factors precipitating reinfarction are hypoxaemia, dehydration, increased metabolic demands, hypercoagulability and acute starvation.

Ultimately the heart fails if its ability to contract continues to decline.

Heart failure results in poor peripheral perfusion, reducing the efficiency of all organs.

*Assessment*
Pulses, blood pressure
Core/surface temperature difference
Urine output
Cerebral status

*Preparation*
Treat heart failure if present
Treat aggravating factors, e.g. obesity, hypertension
Specific therapy as indicated
(See p 45 for summary of the pathophysiology of myocardial oxygen flux)

*Management*
1. Preoxygenation
2. Careful, gentle induction of anaesthesia (avoid relative overdose by careful attention to rate of injection)
3. Topical local anaesthetic to vocal cords and upper trachea (blood pressure, heart rate and dysrhythmias are reduced)
4. ECG monitoring

AVOID
Hypoxia and hypercarbia at all times
Shivering (muscle oxygen demand ↑, cardiac output ↑, myocardial oxygen demand ↑, oxygen supply unchanged → HYPOXAEMIA)
Agents likely to depress the myocardium without reducing the workload, e.g. beta blockers
Excessive sympathetic activity
'Light' anaesthesia
Rapid changes in blood volume

**2. Inadequate preload**

*Causes*
Low blood volume
    Renal failure (post dialysis)
    Inadequate fluid intake
    Excessive fluid loss (vomiting, diarrhoea, haemorrhage)
Phaeochromocytoma
Massive vasodilation
    Gm −ve septicaemia
    Amniotic fluid embolism

Vena caval obstruction
  Supine hypotensive syndrome
  An absolute hypovolaemia will lead to a low central venous
pressure, as will a normal blood volume occupying a large vascular
capacity, as when there is massive peripheral vasodilation leading
to stasis or pooling of blood.

*Problems*
Hypotension
Poor perfusion

*Assessment*
Heart rate, blood pressure, CVP, PCWP.
Core/surface temperature difference
Urine output

*Preparation*
Infusion of appropriate fluids to improve perfusion under close
central venous pressure monitoring

**Table 1** Relative merits of crystalloids, colloids, plasma and blood

| Solution | Adverse reactions | Circulatory half-life (depending upon capillary) integrity) |
|---|---|---|
| 0.9% saline | – | |
| Haemaccel | + | 30 min |
| Gelofusine | + | 1½ h |
| Dextran 70 | + | 3½ h |
| Plasma protein fraction | – | hours |
| Blood | + | days |

*Management*
1. No premedication if peripheral perfusion poor (ventilatory and
   cardiovascular depression may result leading to a further
   reduction in tissue oxygenation)
2. Ketamine/pancuronium technique
   In the absence of maximal adrenergic drive both ketamine and
   pancuronium cause an increase in heart rate and blood
   pressure. Other agents have been described as causing minimal
   cardiovascular changes—neuroleptanaesthesia, an
   opiate/droperidol combination
3. Infuse fluids to produce, or maintain the production of, urine.

AVOID
A sudden fall in peripheral resistance or blood volume
High intrathoracic pressures—reduces venous return

### 3.  Excessive afterload

*Cause*
—severe hypertension
—severe coarctation

*Management*
Heart failure associated with hypertension is an indication for acute therapy. Frusemide and methyldopa are drugs of choice; hydrallazine and prazosin, vasodilators, are also effective in reducing the afterload. Other drugs that have been used are sodium nitroprusside, labetalol, diazoxide, clonidine and guanethidine
Coarctation may need urgent surgery if heart failure is present

### 4.  Inefficient heart rate (<40 or >160/min in the adult)

*Causes of tachycardia*
Apprehension/anxiety ⎫
Pyrexia              ⎪
Pain                 ⎬ Usually sinus rhythm
Hypovolaemia         ⎪
Hypercarbia          ⎭
Ischaemic heart disease
   Fast atrial fibrillation
   Flutter
   Ventricular tachycardia
Endocrine disorders
   Thyrotoxicosis
   Phaeochromocytoma
Pharmacologically-induced
   Parasympatholytic agents
   Sympathomimetic agents

*Causes of bradycardia*
Physiological sinus bradycardia
Ischaemic heart disease
   Heart block
Pharmacologically induced
   Digoxin
   Beta adrenergic receptor blockade

*Problems*
The common outcome is that of poor perfusion, as a tachycardia allows insufficient time for adequate ventricular filling and a bradycardia causes a fall in cardiac output because the stroke volume cannot compensate for the low heart rate.

*Management of common dysrhythmias*

| | |
|---|---|
| Sinus bradycardia | Atropine |
| Sinus tachycardia | Beta adrenergic blockers |
| Supraventricular arrhythmia | Beta blockers, verapamil, amiodarone |
| Ventricular arrhythmia | Lignocaine, beta blockers, procainamide, quinidine, bretylium |

*Assessment*
Assess state of poor perfusion as above

*Preparation*
Adjust dose of pharmacological agents if considered responsible, or change the drug
Treat underlying pathology if possible
Cardiac pacing may be necessary
   Complete heart block
   Stokes Adams attacks

*Management*
Minimise changes in blood volume and peripheral resistance by using appropriate agents in the correct dose and injection rate and by adequate fluid replacement
CARE with diathermy/pacing—check compatibility—an external pacing device should be available

Note:
   'Demand' pacemakers are inhibited by impulses of frequency within the normal physiological range.
   'Fixed rate' pacemakers may trigger an R-on-T arrhythmia in patients whose myocardium is irritable—this may occur during anaesthesia (multiple ventricular ectopics, ventricular tachycardia or ventricular fibrillation).
   Diathermy can totally inhibit a pacemaker, or turn a demand unit into one of fixed rate. Use of diathermy within 15 cm of the electrode or unit may destroy it.
1. The patients pulse should be monitored continuously
2. The indifferent diathermy pad should be as far away as possible from the pacemaker
3. A defibrillator and external pacing device should be at hand

AVOID
Agents likely to make the dysrhythmia worse,
e.g.  atropine in patients with tachycardia
      halothane in patients with bradycardia

### Failure of oxygenation

*Causes*
Rt – Lt shunts (cyanotic congenital heart disease)
    Fallot's tetralogy
    Ebsteins anomaly
    Tricuspid atresia
    Transposition of great vessels
    Pulmonary stenosis and atrial septal defect
    Anomalous venous drainage
    Eisenmenger's syndrome
Pulmonary congestion
    Mitral stenosis
    Left ventricular failure

*Problems*
Hypoxia (heart failure and arrhythmias)
Pulmonary hypertension. This may occur naturally or may result from a Blalock procedure to improve oxygen saturation in the severely cyanosed patient.
A systemic/pulmonary shunt is created. Pulmonary hypertension is common in longstanding mitral stenosis, VSD and left ventricular failure.

*Assessment*
Clinical history and examination
Exercise tolerance
Cardiac catheterisation and angiography

*Preparation*
Treat heart failure if present
Control dysrhythmias
Antibiotic cover to protect against sub-acute bacterial endocarditis

*Management*
1. Sedative premedication without ventilatory depression
2. Preoxygenation
3. ECG monitoring
4. Smooth, gentle induction of anaesthesia

AVOID
Agents likely to change the haemodynamic state, ketamine being a good example in that it raises pulmonary artery pressure
High intrathoracic pressures

## Disorders of vasomotor control
An inability of the peripheral vasculature to respond to changes occurring elsewhere in the system renders the patient vulnerable.
1. Fixed tone
2. Variable tone
3. Chronic increased tone

### 1. Fixed tone
*Cause*—arteriosclerosis

*General approach*
Myocardial depressants should be avoided, as should sudden changes in posture. Electrocardiographic monitoring is essential.
   Care should be taken to avoid trauma to the skin as healing may be impaired by the poor peripheral circulation.

### 2. Variable tone
—Spinal lesion
—autonomic neuropathy—diabetes, tetanus
—phaeochromocytoma, p 70
—carcinoid, p 71

*General approach*

Spinal cord lesions:
There may be an imbalance in vasomotor tone, in the past epidural local anaesthetic block has been used to improve the circulation in patients with poliomyelitis.
Autonomic reflexes may certainly be obtunded and care should be taken to minimise the cardiovascular fluctuations that may occur.

Autonomic neuropathy:
Patients with longstanding diabetes may develop an autonomic neuropathy. This results in less fine control of the blood pressure and care should be taken during anaesthesia to avoid excess fluid loss as compensatory changes are less effective. There is an increased risk of acute cardiorespiratory death during and after surgery.

### 3. Chronic increased tone
Increase in arteriolar tone may be brought about by a variety of conditions.

*Essential hypertension*
The aetiology of essential hypertension is debated, but it is thought that the primary defect is a renal difficulty in excreting sodium. The blood volume would expand were it not for an increase in a circulating substance that inhibits sodium reabsorption in the

tubules. A sodium transport inhibitor in the circulation however also effects other tissues, smooth muscle being no exception responds by an increase in tone. This increase in tone may become permanent.

*Reno-vascular disease (renal artery stenosis), (p 102)*
*Toxaemia of pregnancy*
*Conn's syndrome*

### General management of the patient with hypertension

1. Control hypertension with beta-adrenergic receptor blockade and other anti-hypertensive agents
2. X-ray chest—heart size, left ventricular failure, aortic coarctation.
   ECG—evidence of left ventricular failure and/or ischaemic heart disease
   Blood electrolytes
3. Normal premedication
4. Monitor CVP, BP, and ECG.
5. Preoxygenation
6. Neuroleptanaesthesia
   $N_2O/O_2$, Fentanyl/Droperidol, Topical local anaesthetic to vocal cords and upper trachea
7. Endotracheal intubation
8. IPPV at normocapnia
9. No pressor agents
10. No myocardial depressants such as halothane

## APPENDIX

### Myocardial $O_2$ consumption
Oxygen consumption can be of several categories
1. Basal $O_2$ demand
2. Heart rate ↑ . . . consumption ↑
3. Contractility ↑ . . . consumption ↑
4. Intraventricular pressure/size of ventricle ∝ wall tension
   tension ↑ . . . consumption ↑
   Thus if the intraventricular pressure is raised then
   . . . consumption ↑

### Myocardial $O_2$ supply
1. During diastole
   The $O_2$ supply is proportional to blood flow which is proportional to the (coronary artery filling pressure/resistance) multiplied by time.

   Diastolic time ↑ . . . $O_2$ supply ↑
   Diastolic time ↓ . . . $O_2$ supply ↓

   Therefore, if the heart rate rises, then oxygen delivery falls.

2.  Local vasodilator metabolites $\rightarrow$ vasodilation $\rightarrow$ $O_2$ supply $\uparrow$

AVOID hypertension ...... intraventricular
pressure $\uparrow$ ........................... $O_2$ supply $\downarrow$
AVOID hypotension ..... coronary artery filling
pressure $\downarrow$ ........................... $O_2$ supply $\downarrow$
AVOID tachycardia ....... $O_2$ demand $\uparrow$ ........................ $O_2$ supply $\downarrow$
AVOID hypoxia ................................................................. $O_2$ supply $\downarrow$

## HAEMATOLOGICAL DISORDERS

Blood disorders have FOUR important functional components of
interest to anaesthetists.
Oxygen carriage
Acute haemolysis of red cells
Haemostasis
Increased risk of thrombosis

### Oxygen carriage
Oxygen flux = Cardiac output $\times$ $C_aO_2$
$= \dot{Q}_T \times [(S_aO_2 \times 1.34 \times Hb) + (P_AO_2 \times$ Sol. Coeff. of $O_2$
in plasma)]
Oxygen consumption = Cardiac output $\times$ $(C_aO_2 - C_vO_2)$
   1.  The effects of cardiac output are dealt with under
cardiovascular disturbances (p 36).
   2.  The saturation of haemoglobin with oxygen is determined by
many factors, many of them being of respiratory or
cardiac/cardiovascular origin ($V_A/Q_C$ abnormalities or true shunts)
and these are therefore dealt with in those sections (pp 32, 43)
   Saturation is also determined by other factors.
Factors affecting the affinity of the haemoglobin for oxygen.
   2.3 DPG (see principles of transfusion p 122) $\uparrow$  Rt. shift
   pH                                                                   $[H]^+$ $\uparrow$ Rt. shift
   Temperature rise                                              $\uparrow$ Rt. shift
   Haemoglobinopathies p 47
   Carbon monoxide poisoning p 173
   3.  Haemoglobin concentration is a major component of oxygen
transport and there are many causes of abnormal haemoglobin
levels.

*Causes of anaemia*
Reduced erythropoiesis
   Aplastic anaemia (various types)
   Leukaemia
   Renal disease
Disordered cellular development
   Vitamin $B_{12}$ deficiency
   Folic acid deficiency

Reduced erythrocyte lifespan
    Haemolysis
        Autoimmune disease
        Haemoglobinopathies
        Drug induced
        Transfusion reaction
Haemorrhage
Plasma expansion

*Management of the anaemic patient*
A haemoglobin of about 11 g. $dl^{-1}$ is considered to provide optimal oxygen delivery. Although the oxygen-carrying capacity is reduced, total flow is increased and this results in a net increase in oxygen delivery.

If the haemoglobin concentration falls below 5 g.$dl^{-1}$ hypoxaemia is difficult to detect.

Transfusion should normally be considered if the [Hb] is below 10 g.$dl^{-1}$; this should be carried out at least 24 h preoperatively to allow time for the regeneration of adequate levels of 2.3. DPG.

*Causes of polycythaemia*
Chronic hypoxia
Dehydration
Polycythaemia Vera

*Management of the polycythaemic patient*
A [Hb] of $> 18$ g.$dl^{-1}$ is associated with a rise in blood viscosity such that intravascular thrombosis is more likely. Venesection with appropriate colloid fluid replacement may be carried out. The polycythaemic patient may appear cyanosed, even when oxygen carriage is adequate.

**Acute haemolysis of red cells**

Transfusion reactions
Haemoglobinopathies
    Sickle cell syndromes
        Sickle cell trait            HbA + HbS (<50%)
        Sickle cell anaemia          HbS + HbS (90–95%)   (5–10% HbF)
        Sickle cell HbC disease      HbS + HbC (50:50)
        Sickle cell thallassaemia    HbS + Thall
These conditions are inherited according to basic Mendelian laws.
     A S     x     A S
 A A     A S     A S     S S
Hbs is found most commonly in Central Africans (20% carrier rate), West Indians and in the Northern USA (8% carrier rate). It is also found in Greece, in India and in the Middle East.

HbC is found commonly in northern Ghana—15%.

Beta thallassaemia is found around the Mediterranean, India, China and the Middle East.

'Sickling' depends on the amount of abnormal haemoglobin and the state of deoxygenation.

In general SS and SC sickle at a $Po_2$ of 30–40 mmHg (4–5 kPa) and AS at 20 mmHg (2.5 kPa).

*Problems*
—gelation of HbS . . . sickling . . . haemolytic crisis
—anaemia

*Assessment*
Sickledex test (quick)
Electrophoresis
$P_aO_2$, $S_aO_2$

*Preparation*
Preoperative transfusion if Hb < 5 g.dl$^{-1}$
Exchange transfusion in cases of very major surgery
Treatment of infection if present.

*Management*
Avoidance of hypoxia during and after anaesthesia
Monitoring of oxygen saturation
Avoidance of circulatory stasis, hypothermia and acidosis
The administration of alkalis has been suggested by some workers
Use simple, familiar techniques
Avoid tourniquets if possible

**Haemostasis**
The most common problems are those of haemophilia, thrombocytopaenia, hypofibrinogenaemia, post-transfusion coagulopathy and anticoagulant therapy.

*Haemophilia*
90% of coagulation disorders are due to haemophilia. Factor VIII has to be replaced prior to surgery. Cryoprecipitate is used for this purpose—20–30 ml per bag.
2 units/12 kg body weight is given initially
1 unit/12 kg body weight is given 12-hourly for maintenance.
The biological half life of Factor VIII is 12 h.

*Thrombocytopaenia*
If transfusion is indicated then blood that is less than 12 h old or platelet concentrates should be given. Retinal haemorrhages are

considered a positive indication for transfusion, however if a splenectomy is to be carried out, give the transfusion after excision of the spleen.

*Hypofibrinogenaemia*
This may be the result of disseminated intravascular coagulation, (DIC).

A full clotting 'screen' should be carried out to determine the situation as DIC is a dynamic process and treatment changes depending on the actual state of the process.

The critical fibrinogen level is 100 mg. $dl^{-1}$. A platelet count and the determination of the fibrin degradation products (FDP) may clarify the situation. Excessive coagulation causes a thrombocytopaenia, excessive fibrinolysis increases the FDP.

*Post-transfusion coagulopathy*
1. Platelet deficiency
2. Factor V absent in ACD blood
3. Dilution of the patient's own coagulation factors

*Management*
Clotting 'screen'
Platelets, fresh frozen plasma
Fresh blood

*Anticoagulant therapy*
The prothrombin time should be maintained 1.5–2.5 times the control value. Vitamin K should only be used if absolutely necessary as it may interfere with anticoagulation for a week.

**Increased risk of thrombosis**
Five variables have been shown to identify those patients at risk; euglobulin lysis time, serum concentration of fibrin-related antigen, age, excess weight and varicose veins.

Other preoperative factors have, historically, also been associated with a higher risk of thrombosis; cigarette smoking, polycythaemia and the contraceptive pill.

The type of surgery, gynaecological in particular, and postoperative immobility have also been included in the list of factors predisposing to deep vein thrombosis and pulmonary embolism.

*Management*
Lose excess weight
Stop smoking
Stop taking the contraceptive pill for at least 3 months, (the risk of thrombosis has obviously to be set against the risk of pregnancy)

The use of devices to enhance venous blood flow in the legs,
(inflatable boots, mechanical flexion/extension of the foot)
Early ambulation
The use of prophylactic low dose subcutaneous heparin has to be
weighed against the associated increased risk of bleeding from
such therapy. It is likely that the use of a predictive index of risk,
and to treat only those at risk, is the future ideal solution.

## RENAL DISEASE

There are TWO main aspects of acute renal disease, they are
1. Failure of correct osmole excretion
2. Failure of correct water excretion
1. and 2. may co-exist.

Incorrect osmole excretion {too much—nephrotic syndrome
too little—renal tubular dysfunction

Incorrect water excretion { too much { high output renal failure
Diabetes insipidus
too little—low output renal failure

*Problems*
The problems associated with renal disease can be divided into
three groups, pathophysiological, infective and pharmacokinetic.

## Pathophysiological

*1. Anaemia* (p 46)
The anaemia secondary to renal disease is not perfectly
understood, it is thought to be partially due to a disordered
haemopoietin secretion

*2. Acidosis/electrolyte imbalance* (p 52)
Both acidosis and electrolyte imbalance result from the kidneys'
inability to control the passive or active absorption of ions from the
tubules. Acid/base control is taken over by the lungs.

*3. Dysrhythmias* (p 42)
The dysrhythmias associated with renal disease are those that are
normally associated with potassium disturbances.

*4. Abnormal blood volume* (p 39)
Untreated renal failure leads to an increase in blood volume
whereas the recently dialysed patient may be severely
hypovolaemic.

## Infective
Patients with renal failure are particularly susceptible to hepatitis B
infection, especially those that have undergone haemodialysis.

Routine screening for the hepatitis B surface antigen (HBsAG) is not the norm but it should be considered in those patients are risk and precautions should be taken; if found to be positive, gown up, wear surgical gloves, wear goggles and incinerate all material contaminated with blood or body fluids.

**Pharmacokinetic**
Tissue affinity for drugs may be altered and their binding to plasma proteins is changed. A smaller dose of thiopentone is required to induce sleep in the patient with renal failure than in the normal patient. Only infrequently does hypoproteinaemia increase the unbound active form of the drug.

Prolonged apnoea following suxamethonium administration occurs, this is particularly associated with haemodialysis—there is a relative lack of pseudocholinesterase.

If more than 50% of a drug is excreted through the kidneys then dosage adjustment is necessary according to the glomerular filtration rate.

An ideal drug in renal failure should—
a. not be nephrotoxic
b. < 30% excreted through the kidney
c. no active metabolites
d. unaffected by protein levels

*Assessment*
Clinical history and examination
Full blood count
Urea and electrolytes
Australia antigen
Plasma proteins

*Preparation*
Consider transfusion
There is still considerable debate about the wisdom of pre-operative transfusion in the patient with chronic renal failure as immunological and haematological problems may result
Identify acceptable electrolyte limits
For the patient on regular dialysis electrolyte control should be good; less ideal values may have to be accepted in those in urgent need of surgery and not on dialysis

**Management of the patient with renal disease**
The management of the renal patient has two aims
a. To perform anaesthesia successfully with the problems described above, physiological and pharmacological
b. To avoid causing further derangement to impaired renal function

## 1. Renal blood flow must be maintained

Anaesthesia abolishes autoregulation thus if the blood pressure falls below 80 mm Hg renal blood flow (RBF) will fall, glomerular filtration decreases and urine output drops.

Inhalational agents ...................... RBF ↓ 40% ⎱ depends on the
Thiopentone/$N_2O$/relaxant ........... RBF ↓ 30% ⎰ agent and the dose
Spinal anaesthesia ........................ RBF ↓ proportional to fall in
arterial pressure

## 2. Antidiuretic hormone secretion should be minimised

Barbiturates ......................... ADH secretion does not increase
Narcotics ............................. ADH secretion does not increase
   (High dose narcotic analgesics impair the ADH response to stress)
Phenothiazines .................... ADH secretion falls

AVOID
Fluorinated ethers
   Fluorine concentrations rise following biotransformation of the agent, and these levels may be increased if the agent is given in high concentrations for a prolonged period of time or if enzyme induction has occurred.
   The result of excess free fluorine ions is to produce an ADH resistant polyuria which then becomes an oliguria and urea and potassium ultimately rise.
   For methoxyflurane the recommended dose is 2 MAC hours. (MAC—minimum alveolar concentration of the agent to produce an absence of response to a standard surgical stimulus in 50% of the population)
E.g.  0.16% for 2 hours
      0.32% for 1 hour

   These figures can only be accepted as crude guidelines. Enflurane and isoflurane may present similar problems if enzyme induction exists.

## Assessment of fluid and electrolyte balance

*Extra-cellular fluid volume* (ECF)
Decrease:    Loss of fluid into the intestinal tract
             Renal losses
             Burns
             Osmotic diuresis
             Addison's disease
             Phaeochromocytoma
Increase:    Excessive administration of fluids
             Renal failure
             Congestive cardiac failure

Hepatic cirrhosis
Cushing's disease
Assessment: Clinical history
BP, heart rate, pulse volume
Fullness of veins
Central venous pressure, oedema
Urinary output/fluid balance
Chest X-ray
Treatment: Treat causal process
Fluid administration dependent upon the fluid
balance figures and upon the result of the dynamic
testing of the central venous pressure

*Tonicity*
Decrease: Excess water load (5% dextrose)
Congestive cardiac failure
$K^+$ depletion ($Na^+$ replaces intra-cellular $K^+$)
Excess ADH production
Liver disease
Increase: Inadequate water intake
Excessive losses, e.g.
diabetes insipidus
Assessment: Clinical history and examination
Electrolyte changes are small initially in states of
water intoxication, decreased tonicity, but later the
$[Na^+]$ falls to $<135$ mmol.$1^{-1}$

℞ fluid restriction

Blood volume is well maintained initially in states of
dehydration, increased tonicity but later the [Hb] and
PCV rise, and urine output falls.

℞ 5% dextrose

*Potassium concentration*
Decrease: Vomiting, diarrhoea
Diuretics
Steroid therapy (Cushing's disease)
Diuretic phase of renal failure
Renal tubular acidosis
Villous papilloma
Aldosteronism (Conn's syndrome)
Assessment: Urea and electrolytes
Fluid balance
Treatment: Check that the urine output is satisfactory, then
administer parenteral potassium.

$= <20$ mmol. $hr^{-1}$ or $= <200$ mmol. $day^{-1}$

| | |
|---|---|
| Increase: | Failure of excretion |
| | Acidosis |
| | Spironolactone |
| | Addison's disease |
| Assessment: | Clinical history |
| | Urea and electrolytes |
| | Creatinine |
| | pH |
| | fluid balance |
| Treatment: | Glucose 50 g |
| | Soluble insulin 24 units |
| | 100 ml NaHCO$_3$ 8.4% |
| | Calcium gluconate 10 ml of 10% |
| | Resonium A |
| | Peritoneal dialysis |
| | Haemodialysis |

(A urinary [Na$^+$] > 30 mmol.l$^{-1}$ and a urinary urea concentration of > 1.1 g.dl$^{-1}$ is suggestive of intrinsic renal failure)

## LIVER DYSFUNCTION

There are FOUR functional aspects to liver dysfunction that are of particular interest to the anaesthetist.
1. Jaundice
2. Increased risk of bleeding
    Failure of coagulation
    Portal hypertension
3. Failure of detoxication
4. Australia antigen (hepatitis B surface antigen [HBsAg])

Increased haemoglobin degradation ⟶
Obstructive liver disease ⟶ } Jaundice

Hepatocellular disease
Coagulation defects
Reduced detoxication
Portal hypertension
Australia antigen [HBsAg]

### Jaundice

*Causes*
Increased haemoglobin degradation
    Haemolysis
    Resorption of haematoma
Obstructive liver disease
    Cholelithiasis
    Cholestasis
    Cancer of the head of pancreas

Hepatocellular disease
  Hepatitis
  Cirrhosis
  Poisoning

**Haemorrhage**
Coagulation defects  —reduction in production of coagulation
                        proteins
Oesophageal varices—may rupture spontaneously, or as a result of
                     trauma, nasogastric intubation

**Failure of detoxication**
Choice of drugs and dosages difficult
The effect of a drug in hepatic disease is not very predictable as
there is considerable overlap between the doses required for the
patient with liver disease and the normal population.

**Risk of hepatitis B**
Take precautions if HBsAg positive, p 123

**Management of the patient with liver disease:**

*Assessment*
Clinical history and examination
Drug history
Liver function tests
Plasma proteins
Serum urea and electrolytes
Coagulation 'screen'
Blood ammonia
Australia antigen 'screen'

*Preparation*
Vitamin K therapy if abnormal prothrombin time
Platelets if required
Transfusion if anaemic
Pre-induction infusion of mannitol (bladder catheterisation)
Precautions against AA (HBsAg) contamination
    The anaesthetic management of the patient with liver disease
should be such that further liver dysfunction is minimised.

*1. Premedication*
Care should be taken with opiates, halve the dose, as excretion may
be halved. Benzodiazepines differ in their pharmokinetic
profiles—oxazepam excretion is unchanged; however the dosage
of diazepam should be reduced.

## 2. Induction

If the patient has obstructive jaundice a mannitol infusion should be set up. It is thought that in obstructive jaundice toxins are absorbed from the gut, and not removed by the liver, and it is the concentration of these toxins in the kidney that may be the causative agent in the renal failure that is termed the 'hepato-renal syndrome'. Diuretics, by increasing tubular flow, dilute these toxins. Catheterisation is necessary. The patients most at risk are those with bilirubin concentrations of >140 $\mu$mol.l$^{-1}$. (In addition, diuretics protect the kidney from hypoxic damage, as they reduce the metabolic work that the tubular cells perform.)

Intravenous barbiturates are satisfactory for induction of anaesthesia but they may accumulate if repeated doses are given.

The dose of suxamethonium required may be less because of the lower levels of pseudocholinesterase.

## 3. Care with nasogastric tubes if oesophageal varices are suspected.

## 4. Maintenance

The dose of non-depolarising drugs may need to be large to produce effective relaxation.

Liver dysfunction does not affect the duration of action of inhalational agents as elimination is predominantly via the lungs.

## AVOID

Agents that are predominantly broken down in the liver
Prolonged fasting—as the glycogen depleted liver is at greater risk from the toxic effects of pharmacological agents
Hypotension—poor perfusion leading to hypoxia enhances the toxicity of other agents
Enzyme induction—increased metabolism of drugs leads to an increase in the concentration of toxic free radicals
Known hepatotoxic agents

## Jaundice following general anaesthesia and surgery

There is some epidemiological evidence to suggest that multiple anaesthetics/operations over a relatively short period carry a higher incidence of post-operative jaundice than in other surgical patients.

There has been a tendency in recent years to implicate halothane as a causal agent in this relationship. Despite extensive studies designed to identify halothane and its biodegradation products as hepatotoxic, no certain involvement has been confirmed.

Hypotension, hypoxaemia and hypercarbia can all lead to liver dysfunction and therefore these side effects should be minimised in all general anaesthetic procedures.

It is likely that a combination of circumstances—perhaps anaerobic reductive biodegradation of halothane and the combination of the resultant metabolites with protein, may provoke liver failure in a patient with a genetic 'immunological' predisposition. The entity of 'halothane hepatitis' if it exists is extremely rare.

In the case of the necessity to give multiple anaesthetics over a short period (2 monthly intervals) it is nonetheless wise to administer an agent other than halothane from a 'halothane-free' anaesthetic machine. However, the possibly increased morbidity arising from the use of alternative agents must be weighed against the rare possibility of liver damage arising from the use of halothane.

## DISORDERS OF THE BRAIN, SPINAL CORD, NERVES AND MUSCLE

### Central nervous system
Disorders of the central nervous system can be divided into two groups:
1. Where the cooperation of the patient is limited by their intellectual or psychological defects
   Mental retardation / dementia / confusion
   Psychiatric disorders
2. Where there is an intracranial disease process that requires special management
   Epilepsy
   Raised intracranial pressure
   Cerebral aneurysm
   Parkinsonism
   Deranged blood/brain barrier

### Mental retardation/dementia/confusion

*Causes*
Many idiopathic syndromes
Cerebral dysfunction due to
Hypoxia
Hypoglycaemia
Hypercarbia
Uraemia
Hepatic failure, etc
Cerebral damage due to
Head injury
Infection
Inborn errors of metabolism

*Problems*
Possible lack of cooperation
Concomitant pathology associated with many of the conditions.
   Congenital heart disease
   Endocrine disturbance

*Management*
1. Parenteral premedication is best avoided in the uncooperative patient. An oral tranquilliser is probably best but heavy sedation may be desirable in the grossly disturbed patient.
2. Patients with an organic confusional state are not improved by the administration of drugs; however drugs that are completely metabolised or eliminated quickly are the least likely to cause problems.

## Psychiatric disorders
Most anaesthetic-related problems are associated with drug therapy (p 23).
a. Tricyclic antidepressants
b. Monoamine oxidase inhibitors
c. Lithium

## Epilepsy

*Causes*
Idiopathic
Cerebral trauma or surgery
Tumours
Drug therapy

*Problems*
Induction of enzymes by phenobarbitone, and to a lesser extent by phenytoin, may increase the toxicity of other drugs. The degradation of methoxyflurane is enhanced and thus the concentration of the metabolites is increased.
Competition for degradation pathways may increase the concentration of circulating drugs, for example phenytoin by diazepam.

*Management*
It is important to know the degree of control and frequency of attacks.
Specific drug therapy, phenobarbitone, phenytoin, and diazepam for grand mal, ethosuximide and troxidone for petit mal.
Premedication with drugs with anticonvulsant properties—diazepam, for example, see note above.
Induction and maintenance of anaesthesia with drugs with inherent anticonvulsant properties.
Avoid drugs likely to increase the excitability of the cerebral cortex (ketamine, methohexitone, enflurane, ether, althesin, propanidid and methoxyflurane).
There is some evidence that there may be an increased sensitivity to non-depolarising agents in those patients on phenytoin.

**Raised intracranial pressure** (ICP)

*Causes*
Trauma/oedema
Tumour
Hydrocephalus

*Assessment*
Clinical history and examination
Optic fundi—papilloedema
Intracranial pressure monitoring p 150

*Preparation*
Steroids                    } Reduces oedema and therefore reduces
Fluid restriction          } pressure
Osmotic diuretics        }
Ventricular drainage      Removes CSF—reduces pressure

*Management*
Avoid depressant premedication    } $P_a co_2$ normal or low
No coughing or straining            } Venous pressure minimal
Perfect airway (armoured tube)     } Cerebral perfusion pressure
Adequate ventilation (IPPV)         } lowered
Minimal expiratory resistance     }
Blood pressure not elevated        }

↓

Reduces cerebral blood
volume    ↓

Reduces intracranial
pressure
($P_a co_2 < 20$ mmHg (2.5 kPa) leads to cerebral
vasoconstriction—hypoxia. A mean BP $< 60$ mmHg reduces
cerebral blood flow such that ischaemia is possible)

Minimal concentrations of volatile anaesthetic agents are used, high concentrations cause cerebral vasodilation and thus increase intracranial blood volume and hence intracranial pressure.

**Cerebral aneurysm**

*Problems*
'Steal' and 'inverse steal'

Damaged brain vasculature does not respond to metabolites in the same way as intact brain. If the $P_a co_2$ is raised the normal brain vasculature dilates and 'steals' blood flow from the damaged area. Conversely hypocapnia leads to vasoconstriction of the normal vasculature and the damaged area is preferentially perfused. Avoid extremes.

A bleed from an aneurysm leads to spasm, and an area of cerebral ischaemia. Hypotension should be avoided as this may aggravate the hypoxia.

Hypertension should be avoided as a further bleed may result.

The intracranial pressure should be maintained so that the aneurysm is not unsupported.

A smooth anaesthetic with cardiovascular stability is required.

*Assessment*
Clinical presentation
Computerised axial tomography
Carotid angiography

## Parkinsonism

*Problems*
Spasticity leading to limitation of mobility.

*Management*
The management of patients with Parkinson's disease revolves around the reduction of the spasticity by drug therapy, levo-dopa (p 24); this facilitates mobility and clearing the chest of secretions by allowing greater activity.

## Deranged blood/brain barrier
Meningitis/encephalitis
Multiple sclerosis

*Problems*
Drugs pass to the brain in concentrations that are toxic, e.g. local anaesthetic concentration threshold for convulsions is lowered.

*Management of the patient with multiple sclerosis:*
Assessment:  Note the natural history of the patient's disease
             Determine if the patient suffers with epilepsy: there is an increased incidence
             Respiratory function tests
Preparation: Any infection should be treated vigorously as pyrexia is associated with relapse
             Subcutaneous heparin should be given as there is increased platelet 'stickiness'
Anaesthesia: AVOID atropine—it may cause a rise in temperature
             Diazepam premedication is safe
             AVOID suxamethonium—[K$^+$] may rise and cause arrhythmias
             Non-depolarising muscle relaxants should be used with caution: use a low dose
             ? prophylactic use of anti-pyretics
             LA and spinal techniques are best avoided

**Disorders of the spinal cord and peripheral nerves**
Anaesthetic-orientated problems associated with diseases of the
spinal cord and peripheral nerves are of three types—
cardiovascular stability, potassium release associated with the use
of suxamethonium and respiratory inadequacy.

*Cardiovascular stability* (p 44)
Poliomyelitis—unstable
Multiple sclerosis—unstable
Traumatic cord transection—unstable

*Stability of serum potassium levels following the use of
suxamethonium*
poliomyelitis—stable
multiple sclerosis—unstable
traumatic cord transection—unstable
polyneuropathy—unstable

*Respiratory involvement* (p 34)
Adequacy of ventilation is dependent upon the level at which cord
damage has occurred or which peripheral nerves are involved.

**Neuromuscular disorders**
The functional importance of the neuromuscular disorders can be
described by their effect on muscle power, and thus on respiratory
ventilatory ability, and also their response to the various drugs
used to block the neuromuscular junction or alter muscle tone.
Respiratory inadequacy (p 34)
Abnormal response to neuromuscular blocking agents

*1. Depolarising agents* (suxamethonium)
Atypical cholinesterase            —extended duration of blockade
Myasthenia gravis                  —recovery occurs within minutes
                                     but may be incomplete
Myasthenic syndrome                —extremely sensitive
Dystrophia myotonica               —myotonia increased
Progressive muscular dystrophy—a small dose should be given
                                     and its effect noted

*2. Non-depolarising agents*
Myasthenia gravis                  —extreme sensitivity
Myasthenic syndrome                —extreme sensitivity
Dystrophia myotonica               —neuromuscular transmission is
                                     blocked but myotonia may
                                     persist
Progressive muscular dystrophy—a small dose should be given
                                     and the effect noted

*Atypical cholinesterase*
Enzymatic hydrolysis is the important factor controlling the plasma level of suxamethonium, less than 5% of the injected dose reaches the neuromuscular junction.

96.2% of the population are the 'normal' heterozygote and hydrolyse suxamethonium rapidly, 3.8% are heterozygote and hydrolysis takes 5–10 minutes. 1 in 2800 is the abnormal homozygote and hydrolysis is very prolonged.

There are Dibucaine and fluoride 'resistant' genes and a silent gene.

Prolonged apnoea is best managed by mechanical ventilation with sedation until spontaneous recovery occurs. The use of anticholinesterases in the final stages of recovery, or fresh blood, is not normal practice.

*Myasthenia gravis*
Autoimmune reduced sensitivity to acetylcholine
Assessment: Response to anticholinesterases
            Pulmonary function tests/chest X-ray
Preparation: Anticholinesterase treatment is stopped
            pre-operatively if the patient is able to manage—this reduces bronchorrhoea and produces a partial neuromuscular block. Depressant drugs are best avoided.
Anaesthesia: Induction with minimal thiopentone, $N_2O$, $O_2$ and halothane usually allows intubation, and adequate relaxation. Reversal of relaxation may be carried out in the usual way at the termination of the anaesthetic.

## APUD CELL DISORDERS* (Endocrine and neuro-transmitter disorders)

1. Abnormal Glucocorticoid levels $\begin{cases} \text{Excessively high} \\ \text{Potentially inadequate} \end{cases}$

2. Abnormal Glucose level $\begin{cases} \text{Low} \\ \text{High} \end{cases}$ $\begin{cases} \text{Ketotic} \\ \text{Non-ketotic} \end{cases}$

3. Inappropriate Metabolic rate $\begin{cases} \text{High} \\ \text{Low} \end{cases}$

4. Failure of calcium homeostasis $\begin{cases} \text{High calcium} \\ \text{Low calcium} \end{cases}$

5. Abnormal vasoactive 'hormones/transmitters' $\begin{cases} \text{Catecholamines} \\ \text{Kinins} \end{cases}$

*APUD cells are of neuroectoderm origin and secrete amines and peptides, they are found in the pituitary, pancreas, adrenal gland, thyroid, parathyroids and in carcinoid tumours.

## Excessively high glucocorticoid levels

*Causes*
High dose steroid therapy
Cushing's disease

*Problems*
Fluid retention p 52
Potassium depletion p 52
Hypernatraemia p 52
Hypertension p 44
Impaired glucose tolerance p 65
Reduced protein synthesis (poor healing)
Osteoporosis
Muscle weakness

*Assessment*
Adrenal function tests
 Plasma cortisol
 ACTH or Tetracosactrin response
 Response to insulin induced hypoglycaemia
  (Tests afferent and efferent pathways)
 Metapyrone test
  (Tests efferent pathway)

*Preparation*
Treat hypertension, electrolyte imbalance and glucose intolerance.

*Management*
Glucocorticoid supplementation is essential, and in greater doses than normally used (200 mg hydrocortisone 6-hourly) because of the adaptation of tissues to very high levels. Weaning from steroids should be carried out slowly.

## Potentially inadequate glucocorticoid levels

*Causes*
Suppression of adrenal cortex due to steroid therapy
Bilateral adrenalectomy
Addison's disease
 Autoimmune adrenalitis (80% of cases)
 Tuberculosis
 Adrenal haemorrhage, infarction
  Meningococcal septicaemia
 Amyloidosis
Hypopituitarism
 Trauma
 Infection
 Space-occupying lesion

*Problems*
Hypotension
Inability to respond to stressful situations—impaired reflex
circulatory control—hypotension, 'shock'
Weakness
Possible sensitivity to narcotics

*Assessment*
Adrenal function tests
    Pituitary/adrenal axis function tests as above
    High plasma ACTH, low cortisol—primary adrenocortical
    insufficiency
    Check adequacy of other endocrine systems

*Preparation*
Addison's disease—replacement therapy for all zones of the cortex
Secondary adrenal insufficiency—glucocorticoid replacement only
    Glucocorticoid:
                        Cortisol 20 mg 0800 h
                                10 mg 1800 h
    Mineralocorticoid:
                        Fludrocortisone 0.05—0.15 mg daily

*Management*
Additional steroid cover is required during surgery, (100 mg
    hydrocortisone 6-hourly). There is an increased sensitivity to
    narcotics and barbiturates. The benzodiazepines are
    recommended as premedication.

**Low glucose level**

*Causes*
Antidiabetic medication in excess of needs
    Insulin treated diabetics and those on chlorpropramide at risk
Post-alcohol hypoglycaemia
Insulinoma

*Problems*
Severe hypoglycaemia leads to brain damage

*Assessment*
Fasting blood sugar
Glucose tolerance tests
Urinalysis—(if always free of sugar they are at risk)
Hb—monitored to assess adequacy of antidiabetic therapy

*Preparation*
Check control of diabetes
    If on insulin:
        Stabilise on short acting preparation if normally on a long
        acting agent
        Perform fasting blood sugar on day of operation
        Set up an insulin and dextrose infusion to replace usual calorie
        intake prior to theatre
        Arrange operation for the earliest time, although this is not so
        important if the above advice is taken as the patient will be well
        controlled
    If on oral hypoglycaemic agents:
        Stop chlorpropramide 24 h preoperatively

*Management*
Maintain blood sugar using dextrostix as an indicator of correct
management

AVOID
Discontinuation of calorie intake whilst maintaining insulin
treatment
Heavy premedication or anaesthesia—the patient's state of
consciousness should be assessed at the end of the procedure

**High glucose levels**

*Causes*
Untreated or inadequately treated diabetes mellitus
Insulin resistance (found in sick patients)
Insulin antagonism (excess growth hormone)

*Problems*
Acidosis
Hypokalaemia (p 53)

*Assessment*
Blood sugar
Urea and electrolytes
Investigate reason for lack of diabetic control
(infection, other endocrine abnormalities)

*Preparation*
Delay surgery if possible so that the diabetic state can be controlled
Uncontrolled diabetes is a contraindication to anaesthesia/surgery
unless the surgical necessity is great. Alternately, drainage of an
abcess may be fundamental to the management of the diabetes
and thus anaesthesia is necessary.

Ketoacidosis should be brought under control with a regimen of dextrose/insulin/potassium and close biochemical and clinical scrutiny.
Extremely urgent surgery, which cannot be delayed, associated with ketoacidosis and hyperkalaemia has a high mortality.

*Management*
Dextrose/insulin/potassium infusion with biochemical control—monitor intra-operative blood sugar
ECG monitoring
Take precautions against pulmonary aspiration: diabetics are at great risk
Use a balanced anaesthesia technique

AVOID
Underventilation
Ether—produces hyperglycaemia

**High metabolic rate**

*Causes*
Pyrexia
Thyrotoxicosis—excessive production of T3/T4
  *Problems associated with thyrotoxicosis:*
—Enlarged thyroid—possible upper airway compression p 29
—High cardiac output (p 36)
—Excessive adrenergic activity (p 41), tachycardia, dysrthythmias—atrial fibrillation common
—Myopathy
—Possible thyrotoxic crisis

*Assessment*
Clinical history and examination
Isotope uptake ($^{99}$Tc $^{131}$I, $^{132}$I)
T3 and T4 levels
Protein bound iodine
ECG
X-ray of thoracic inlet—to demonstrate tracheal patency

*Preparation*
Specific therapy
Antithyroid medication where indicated (including beta blockers)
Antibiotics/antipyretics/active cooling

*Management*
Specific therapy
Pyrexia —antipyretics, antibiotics if indicated, active
cooling
Thyrotoxicosis—1. Carbimazole ⎱ Blocks binding of iodine to
           Methimazole ⎰ mono and di-iodotyrosine
           Thiouracils
         2. Radio-active iodine (patients over 40 years)
         3. Beta-adrenergic receptor blockade
Atropine is best avoided in pyrexia—sweating, and therefore
heat loss, is decreased. Premedication with phenothiazines is said
to enhance anti-thyroid drugs and reduce thyrotrophin secretion.

General anaesthesia is normally well tolerated in the absence of
heart failure, ECG monitoring however is essential.

An acute surgical emergency may precipitate a state of severe
and uncontrolled thyrotoxicosis termed a thyrotoxic crisis.
a. Hyperpyrexia
b. Confusion, restlessness, delirium, apathy, prostration
c. Tachycardia, atrial fibrillation, cardiac failure
d. Flushing and sweating
e. Vomiting, diarrhoea and abdominal pain
f. Dehydration and ketosis

*Treatment*
Oxygen
Sedation
Fluid and electrolyte replacement
Surface cooling
Sodium iodide (0.5 g i.v. every 4 h)
Carbimazole—for later benefit
Beta-adrenergic blockade
Hydrocortisone should adrenal failure occur
Guanethidine for hypertension
Digitalis for congestive heart failure

**Low metabolic rate**

*Causes*
Hypothermia
Myxoedema

*Problems*
Low cardiac output, low heart rate, poor contractility—myocardial
ischaemia (p 38)
Poor ability to metabolise drugs therefore great sensitivity to them.
Possible pituitary/adrenal hypofunction p 63
Possible polyneuropathy

*Assessment*
Clinical history and examination
Temperature
ECG
Serum electrolytes and blood sugar (inappropriate ADH secretion)
Clotting 'screen'
Thyroid function tests (as above)

*Preparation*
Anaesthesia in the presence of severe myxoedema is associated
with a high mortality. Postpone surgery if possible. Hypothermia
*per se* may protect the patient against acute hypoxia but great care
is needed to avoid further depression of cardiac function.

The myxoedematous patient should be treated with
triiodothyronine (peak effect 48–72 h) in an attempt to return
physiological function to normal although this may lead to
dysrhythmias and heart failure. The ECG must be monitored.

Hydrocortisone is necessary to protect the patient against
adrenocortical insufficiency.

The hypothermic patient should be allowed to regain normal
temperature if there is not need for the hypothermia. Passive
warming techniques are preferable to active 'surface' techniques
(see below); they avoid the danger of burning the patient's skin.

*Management*
1. Premedication is best avoided
2. Use very small doses of drugs and assess their effect with care.
3. Maintain with care the blood volume
4. Monitor the ECG
5. Core and surface temperature (consider active 'central'
   rewarming if core temperature below 30°C)
6. Adjust ventilation to maintain a normal $P_aco_2$ ($CO_2$ solutbility ↑
   as temperature ↓)

AVOID
Overventilation
Large changes in haemodynamics
Large surface/core temperature gradient; it may lead to profound
changes in core temperature if the patient's limbs are moved or
elevated, and this may result in ventricular fibrillation
Damage to skin: if a heated blanket is used then the blanket should
be only 1–2°C above the patient's surface temperature
Chronotropic drugs

*Note*
Infections are common and congestive cardiac failure is easily
precipitated. Myxoedema coma has a mortality of 80% and can be
caused by carbon dioxide retention.

## High calcium levels

*Cause*
Hyperparathyroidism
   Primary—adenoma, hyperplasia, carcinoma
   Secondary to renal failure

*Problems*
Muscle weakness (sensitivity to muscle relaxants)
Spontaneous fractures
Restricted thoracic cavity (p 34)

*Assessment*
Clinical history and examination
Serum calcium level (raised)
Chest X-ray, skeletal survey
ECG
Urea and electrolytes
Radio immune assay of parathormone
Electromyography
Pulmonary function tests

*Preparation*
Calcitonin

*Management*
Anaesthesia is not normally associated with problems specifically related to abnormal calcium levels
Use relaxants cautiously (use nerve stimulator to assess the degree and nature of block)
Take care when moving and posturing the patient; the skeleton may be fragile
Control respiration if respiratory function is poor

## Low calcium levels

*Causes*
Hypoparathyroidism (1% of patients post-thyroidectomy)
Excess citrate (stored blood)
Post-parathyroidectomy for hyperparathyroidism

*Problem*
If calcium ion concentration < 1.25 mmol—tetany
                                      —laryngeal spasm
                                      —cardiac irritability

*Assessment*
Clinical history and examination
Serum calcium concentration low (possible tetany)
Urea and electrolytes
Plasma proteins
Electromyography

*Preparation*
Parathyroid hormone
Calcium
Vitamin D

*Management*
1. Treat hypocalcaemia
2. Use relaxants with care (use nerve stimulator to assess degree and type of block)
3. Monitor ECG
4. ? Cover massive transfusions with additional calcium

AVOID
Hyperventilation—alkalosis decreases ionised calcium
Excess infusion of alkaline fluids

**Phaeochromocytoma**
A chromaffin tissue tumour; hypertension occurs in 90% of cases, it is paroxysmal in 40%.

*Problems*
Sympathetic overactivity
Diminished blood volume
Possible hyperglycaemia

*Assessment*
Clinical history and examination
ECG
Hb or PCV, high values indicate a contracted blood volume
Metanephrine excretion (> 1.3 mg/24 h)
Selective sampling from inferior vena cava to determine tumour sites
Blood sugar

*Preparation*
Alpha-adrenergic receptor blockade (10–14d) with phenoxybenzamine orally
Gradual restoration of blood volume
Beta-adrenergic receptor blockade is also considered of value, it provides background antiarrhythmia cover

*Anaesthesia*
Sedative premedication
Monitor ECG, intra-arterial pressure, CVP
Hypertension is controlled by intermittent phentolamine
(1–5 mgIV) or by the infusion of sodium nitroprusside (SNP). The
systolic blood pressure should be maintained at about 80 mmHg.
(The total dose of SNP should not exceed 0.5 mg.kg$^{-1}$ and the
infusion rate should not exceed 0.01 mg.kg$^{-1}$.min$^{-1}$.

High dosage overloads the metabolic pathway and free cyanide
is formed. Metabolic acidosis occurs as anaerobic metabolism
predominates)

Hypotension is treated by fluid infusion; if this is ineffective a
pressor agent may be necessary: methoxamine, or
metaraminol—these should be used with care.

A neuroleptanaesthesia technique with IPPV is safe.

AVOID
Hypoxia, hypercarbia, histamine release, sympathetic agents,
handling the tumour, fear, stress and pain
Cyclopropane, chloroform, trichloroethylene, ether and
halothane—either because of their sympathetic effects or potential
for cardiac dysrhythmias in the presence of adrenaline
Suxamethonium—fasciculations may cause compression of the
tumour and thus expression of catecholamine

Postoperative morbidity usually due to unresponsive hypo- or
hypertension leading to congestive heart failure or a
cerebro-vascular accident.

**Carcinoid**
(Originally called 'carcinoid' because it ran a more benign course
than other carcinomas)

The secretion of kallikrein (which catalyses the conversion of
kininogen to bradykinin) and 5-hydroxytryptamine (5HT) causes
flushing, diarrhoea and bronchospasm in a small proportion of
patients with the tumour. Triscuspid and pulmonary stenosis may
also occur.

The detoxification of 5HT and bradykinin in the liver cannot take
place when secreted by a metastasis distal to the liver, this is when
symptoms become apparent.

*Problems*
Possible valvular heart disease
Effects of 5HT—variable effect on vascular tone, depends on the
initial tone

BP ↑ if tone low BP ↓ if tone high

—mild hyperglycaemia

Effects of bradykinin—vasodilation and hypotension
                          —increased capillary permeability
                          —bronchoconstriction

*Assessment*
Clinical history and examination
Serum proteins—exchange of tumour for liver may be reflected in
                          a low protein concentration
Blood sugar

*Preparation*
1 hour pre-operatively infuse aprotinin (a kallikrein trypsin inhibitor)
at a rate of 50000 units per hour
Methotrimeprazine (2.5–5.0 mg i.v.) has been suggested as the
anti-5HT drug of choice

*Anaesthesia*
Sedative premedication
Smooth induction/intubation—local anaesthetic to vocal cords and
trachea
Pancuronium is the relaxant of choice
Neuroleptanaesthesia has been advocated because of the anti-5HT
effect of droperidol. Fentanyl or phenoperidine is satisfactory.
Monitor the ECG, intra-arterial pressure, CVP, blood gases and
electrolytes intra-operatively

AVOID
Morphine—releases 5HT
Suxamethonium—fasciculations/raised intra-abdominal pressure
may cause the release of hormone from the tumour
D-tubocurarine—hypotension, histamine release and
bronchoconstriction
Gallamine—tachycardia
Catecholamine vasopressors

## DERMATOLOGICAL PROBLEMS

### Atopy
Eczema, asthma, and hayfever.
   The skin lesions do not present an anaesthetic problem, other
than that the siting of intravenous infusions may be restricted, the
ante-cubital fossa is commonly involved.
   Atopic patients however are thought to be at greater risk from
adverse reactions to drugs solubilised in Cremofor EL.

**Burns** see p 166
**Epidermolysis bullosa**
This is a rare disorder in which blisters form in response to mild trauma to the skin and mucous membranes. Scarring may occur.
Every precaution should be taken to avoid trauma—endotracheal intubation is best avoided. A hydrocortisone soaked swab should be placed between the face and mask and only gentle pressure used to maintain a gas tight fit.
Porphyria is associated with this condition, p 26

## APPENDIX

Index of disease processes with their major 'anaesthesia'-orientated functional defects.

| | |
|---|---|
| Acromegaly | Upper airway problem |
| | Glucose intolerance |
| Acute intermittant | Adverse |
| porphyria: | reaction to certain |
| | drugs |
| Addison's disease: | Low cardiac output |
| | Inability to respond to stress |
| | Low glucose level |
| Allergy: | Adverse reaction to certain |
| | drugs. |
| Aortic incompetence: | Fixed cardiac output |
| Aortic stenosis: | Fixed cardiac output |
| Anaemia: | Reduced oxygen carriage |
| Ankylosing | Upper airway problem |
| spondylitis: | (intubation problem) |
| Anxiety/depression/ | Possible drug interactions |
| psychosis: | Possible reduced ability to |
| | cooperate |
| Atrial | Associated with ischaemic |
| fibrillation/flutter: | heart disease |
| | thyrotoxicosis, rheumatic |
| | heart disease |
| | Low cardiac output |
| | Inadequate contractility |
| | Inefficient heart rate |
| Bronchiectasis: | Lower airway problem |
| | Excess secretions |
| Bronchitis: | Lower airway problem |
| | Excess secretions |

| | |
|---|---|
| Bronchopleural fistula | Lower airway problem |
| | Leak |
| | Excess secretions |
| Bullous disorders: | Skin and mucous membranes at risk |
| Burns: | Possible low cardiac output |
| | Inadequate preload (low blood vol) |
| | Inadequate contractility (electrolyte imbalance) |
| | Reduced oxygen carriage |
| | Increased risk of renal failure |
| | Altered metabolic state |
| | Possible upper airway problems |
| Carcinoid syndrome: | Abnormal vasomotor control |
| | Variable vascular tone |
| Christmas disease: | Disorder of coagulation |
| Congenital heart disease: | Cyanotic |
| | Failure of oxygenation (Right → Left shunt) |
| | Low cardiac output |
| | Inefficient circulation path within the heart |
| | Acyanotic |
| | Excess pulmonary flow may lead to pulmonary hypertension |
| | Low cardiac output |
| | Inadequate contractility |
| Conn's syndrome: | Disorder of electrolyte homeostasis |
| | Possible high cardiac output |
| | Increased preload |
| Cushings disease: | Possible high cardiac output |
| | Increased preload |
| | Glucose intolerance |
| | Disorder of electrolyte homeostasis |
| Diabetes insipidus: | Low cardiac output |
| | Inadequate preload |
| | Disorder of water homeostasis |
| Diabetes mellitus: | Glucose intolerance |
| | Disorder of electrolyte homeostasis |
| Deep vein thrombosis: | Increased risk of thrombosis |

Diffuse intravascular coagulation: Disorder of coagulation

Drug addiction/intoxication: Decreased metabolism of drugs
Australia antigen—hepatitis B

Dystrophia myotonica: Adverse reaction to certain drugs

Emphysema: Lower airway problem
Failure of oxygenation
V/Q abnormalities

Epilepsy: Adverse reaction to certain drugs

Familial periodic paralysis: Disorder of electrolyte homeostasis
Abnormally responsive receptors (neuro-muscular junction)

Haemophilia: Disorder of coagulation

Heart block: Low cardiac output
Inefficient heart rate

Hyperparathyroidism: Disorder of electrolyte homeostasis
Adverse reaction to certain drugs
If longstanding—Skeletal abnormalities
Restricted thoracic cage
Critical ventilatory ability
Renal failure

Hyperpituitarism: See acromegaly, Cushing's syndrome

Hypertension: Abnormal vasomotor control
Chronically increased tone

Hyperthyroidism: High cardiac output
Excess adrenergic activity
Dysrhythmias

Hypoparathyroidism: Disorder of electrolyte homeostasis
Upper airway problem
Laryngeal spasm
Tetany

Hypopituitarism: Low cardiac output
Inadequate preload
Disorder of electrolyte homeostasis
Glucose intolerance—hypoglycaemia
Inability to respond to stress

Hypothermia:                        Low cardiac output
                                        Inefficient heart rate
                                        Reduced contractility
                                        Dysrhythmias
                                    Reduced ability to metabolise
                                        drugs
                                    Reduced ability to respond to
                                        stress
Hypothyroidism:                     Low cardiac output
                                        Inefficient heart rate
                                        Reduced contractility
                                    Reduced ability to metabolise
                                        drugs
                                    Reduced ability to respond to
                                        stress
Intestinal obstruction:             Low cardiac output
                                        Inadequate preload
                                    Disorder of electrolyte
                                        homeostasis
Ischaemic heart                     Low cardiac output
disease:                                Inadequate contractility
                                        Inefficient heart rate
                                            (dysrhythmias)
Jaundice:                           Increased risk of renal failure
Meningitis:                         Increased sensitivity to certain
                                        drugs
                                        Deranged blood/brain
                                            barrier
Mental retardation:                 Possible lack of cooperation
Mitral incompetence:                Fixed cardiac output
                                    Dysrhythmias
Mitral stenosis:                    Fixed cardiac output
                                    Dysrhythmias
Multiple sclerosis:                 Adverse reaction to certain
                                        drugs
                                    Deranged blood/brain barrier
Muscular dystrophy:
Myasthenia gravis:                  Increased sensitivity to certain
                                        drugs
                                    Abnormally responsive
                                        receptors
                                    Critical ventilatory ability
                                    Lower airway problem
                                        Exess secretions (drug
                                            induced)

Myasthenic syndrome: | Increased sensitivity to certain drugs
Abnormally responsive receptors

Osteomalacia: | Skeletal problem

Pagets disease: | Skeletal problem
Abnormal vasomotor control
Chronically decreased peripheral resistance
Heart failure (rare)

Parkinsonism: | Possible drug interactions
Critical ventilatory ability

Pericarditis (constrictive): | Fixed cardiac output
Fixed stroke volume

Peripheral arterial disease: | Abnormal vasomotor control
Fixed tone
(Associated with ischaemic heart disease)

Peripheral neuropathology: | Increased sensitivity to certain drugs
Abnormally responsive receptors
Possible critical ventilatory ability
Possible abnormal vasomotor control
Variable tone

Phaeochromocytoma: | Abnormal vasomotor control
Variable tone ((excess @ adrenergic activity)

Poliomyelitis: | Possible critical ventilatory ability
Possible electrolyte disturbance in the acute stages in association with the use of suxamethonium (hyperkalaemia)

Pneumonia: | High cardiac output
Tachycardia (pyrexia)
Lower airway problem
Excess secretions
Failure of oxygenation
V/Q abnormality

Pneumothorax/cyst/bulla: | Possible critical ventilatory ability

Pulmonary embolism:    Low cardiac output
                       Inadequate preload to left
                       heart
                       Failure of oxygenation
                       $\dot{V}/\dot{Q}$ abnormality
Renal failure:         Variable cardiac output
                       Increased or decreased
                       preload
                       Disorder of electrolyte
                       homeostasis
Rheumatoid arthritis:  Skeletal problems
                       Reduced ventilatory ability
                       Possible inadequate response
                       to stress (secondary to drug
                       therapy)
Scleroderma:           Upper airway problem
                       (intubation difficulty)
                       Possible critical ventilatory
                       ability
Sickle cell disease:   Oxygen carriage disorder
                       Abnormally at risk from
                       haemolysis
Thalassaemia:          Abnormally at risk from
                       haemolysis
Von Willebrand's       Disorder of haemostasis
disease:

# 3. Considerations for procedures requiring anaesthesia

## EMERGENCY SURGERY

### Dangers
Incomplete history including drug therapy/allergy
Incomplete biochemical, cardiological and radiological examination
Patient's condition progressive, not static
Gastric stasis—danger of regurgitation

### Special action to take
Anticipate exaggerated responses to drugs e.g. hypotension
Balance the risk of anaesthesia and surgery against need for
immediate surgery (e.g. stomach probably empty if trauma
occurred 3 h after a meal, however stomach may still be full 24 h
later if trauma occurred immediately after food). Urgent need for
surgery may deny the opportunity to delay surgery and allow time
for spontaneous gastric emptying. The stomach may be emptied by
the use of a stomach tube, nasogastric tube or emetic.
Preoxygenation
Cricoid pressure
Quick intubation

## SURGERY OF THE HEAD AND NECK

### General problems
1. The patency of the airway must be protected—reinforced
   endotracheal tube + dental ring well secured
2. Eyes must be protected—sticky tape, Vaseline gauze or eye pad
3. Intravenous infusions should be sited so that they are easily
   accessible and away from the operating site
4. Blood pressure and ECG monitoring equipment should be
   attached and operational before skin preparation commences
5. Co-axial circuits are useful because they reduce bulk of tubing
6. Integrity of anaesthetic circuit should be easily confirmed even
   when hidden under drapes, e.g. monitoring of expired gas or
   measurement of airway pressure are suitable methods

## ANAESTHESIA FOR NEUROSURGERY

There are general considerations which are common to most intracranial procedures: these include posture, induced hypotension (p 117) and avoidance of air embolism.

### Effect of posture

*Supine.*   The supine position is least likely to upset the cardiorespiratory systems, the isolation of blood in dependent parts is reduced and there is no compression of the abdomen and hence the inferior vena cava (assuming the absence of gross obesity or an intra-abdominal mass).

The alveolar dead space is minimal when horizontal and the risk of gas embolism is low.

*Prone.*   Special attention must be paid to the protection of the eyes and face, and to the positioning of the head and neck. Support must be provided under the chest and pelvis so that the abdomen is not compressed leading to pressure on the inferior vena cava and splinting of the diaphragm. Positive pressure ventilation is mandatory in the prone position for all surgical procedures including neurosurgical.

*Sitting position.*   The cardiovascular system must be carefully monitored during the transition from the horizontal to the sitting position. Pooling of blood occurs in dependent limbs. Air embolism is more likely in the sitting position. Some neurosurgical units use 'G' suits over the lower half of the body to aid central venous filling.

### Gas embolism

Cause

Gas bubbles will enter the circulation if a vessel with an intraluminal pressure lower than atmospheric is held open. This occurs most commonly to vessels in bony channels and to the venous sinuses within the skull.

Effect

A small volume of gas may go unnoticed, although Doppler sensors over the praecordium can detect very small amounts (0.25 ml). Larger volumes cause disturbances in respiratory rhythm and may lead to a complete failure of cardiac output due to the heart's inability to pump froth. Cerebral function can be seriously deranged.

Prophylaxis

The sitting position increases the likelihood of air embolism by producing low venous pressure in the head and neck. The sitting position should be avoided when possible.

Flooding the operation site with saline will prevent the ingress of air, but is difficult for the surgeon; bone wax is used to seal the bone surface. Praecordial monitoring is mandatory in the sitting position. A 'mill-wheel' murmur may be heard through a stethoscope if gas is present in the heart (this is really too late), a Doppler sensor will identify the embolus much earlier. A sudden fall in $F_{ET}CO_2$ may also occur.

Management
The surgical site should be flooded with saline, venous pressure should be increased (tipping the table head down is usually impossible, and very unpopular with the surgeon) by using PEEP or a 'G' suit. The inspired gas should be 100% $O_2$ ($N_2O$ will enlarge the size of air bubbles) and external cardiac compression may be necessary. It is said that gas can be aspirated from the heart via a central venous line. This manoeuvre may be facilitated by turning the patient into the left lateral position so that the right side of the heart is upper most and thereby preventing the gas bubble from passing into the pulmonary circulation. This is difficult. If a major embolus occurs early in the procedure the operation should be abandoned.

**The patient with raised intracranial pressure**

Causes
Increased CSF volume (hydrocephalus)
Increased brain volume (tumour/oedema)
Increased intracranial blood volume (venous congestion/arterial dilatation)
Hypoxaemia and hypercarbia (respiratory obstruction/respiratory depression)
Subarachnoid and extradural haemorrhage
    Cerebral perfusion pressure (mean arterial pressure—CSF pressure) is the most important cardiovascular factor in patients with raised ICP.

Maintenance of cerebral perfusion

AVOID
1. Venous congestion
   coughing/vomiting
   overhydration
   raised intrathoracic pressure
2. Arterial hypotension
   Care with use of vasodepressant drugs
   in the presence of a relative hypovolaemia

3. Cerebral artery vasodilation (ICP ↑ ) due to
   Anaesthetic agents
   a) Halothane
   b) Trichloroethylene
   c) Methoxyflurane
   $P_aCO_2$ ↑
   Hypoxia

Preparation
DEHYDRATE brain tissue by limiting fluid intake and by specific
hyperosmolar agents. The use of mannitol and urea should be
restricted to the period immediately prior to surgery to avoid the
rebound phenomenon leading to a rise in intracranial pressure
associated with the movement of agent into the brain tissue.
   STEROIDS reduce intracranial pressure by reducing oedema
associated with tumours, trauma and hypoxia.
   CSF DRAINAGE—prior to the definitive surgical procedure a
ventricular drain may be inserted to reduce the dangers associated
with severely rised intracranial pressures—optic atropy, nerve
damage and coning of the medulla.

Essential points of management
1. Dehydrating agents
2. Controlled ventilation
3. Avoiding venous congestion
4. Avoiding excessive use of trichloroethylene, halothane and
   methoxyflurane
   Induced hypotension and cooling have been used to facilitate
difficult surgery.

Special postoperative care
1. Ensure that relaxation is reversed and adequate spontaneous
   ventilation is established prior to extubation
2. Monitor CSF pressure (p 150)
3. If ventilation controlled monitor end tidal carbon dioxide
   concentration
4. Monitor neurological function (p 148)

**The patient with normal intracranial pressure**

*Reasons for intracranial surgery*
Cerebral artery aneurysm
Vascular anomaly
Other non-obstructive lesions

*Problems associated with patients with cerebral aneurysms*
Possible hypertension/instability of blood pressure
A flaccid brain (due to dehydration) may remove support from the
aneurysm and cause further bleeding

*Preparation*
Sedation and/or antihypertensives

*Essential points of management*

AVOID
—a rise in $P_aco_2$
—a rise in venous pressure
—hypoxia
—ventilatory obstruction, PEEP
—hypertension
and minimise the use of inhalational agents
   A short period of intense hypotension may be required during the clipping of an aneurysm; this can be achieved using sodium nitroprusside or trimetaphan.

## OPHTHALMIC SURGERY

**Special factors**
1. Control of intraocular pressure (IOP) (normal 25 mmHg).
2. Drugs used in anaesthesia may affect pupil size
3. Oculo-cardiac reflex

1. Many of the factors affecting intracranial pressure, as described above, also affect intraocular pressure.

   IOP ↓ Halothane, morphine, pethidine, barbiturates, mannitol, acetazolamide, pilocarpine, anticholinesterases, non-depolarising muscle relaxants
   IOP ↑ Suxamethonium, ketamine, atropine (not i.v.), coughing, straining, vomiting and hypertension.
2. Miotics: these agents cause constriction of the pupil; in acute glaucoma a reduction in IOP results as the angle of the anterior chamber is cleared of the pupillary muscle.
   Anticholinesterases
   Carbachol, pilocarpine

   Mydriatics: Mydriasis can precipitate acute glaucoma in those patients at risk; intravenous atropine in normal dosage is not a hazard in this respect
   Belladonna alkaloids, atropine, hyoscine, lachesine cyclopentylate
3. Aschner's oculo-cardiac reflex (afferent fibres in ophthalmic branch of trigeminal nerve, efferent fibres in the vagus): Bradycardia and cardiac arrest are associated with traction on the eyeball. The incidence may be reduced by atropine and by drugs with atropine like effects particularly if combined with relaxation, e.g. gallamine.

**Emergency open eye surgery/full stomach/suxamethonium**
Suxamethonium used to facilitate intubation during induction of general anaesthesia may lead to vitreous prolapse. The risk of vomiting, with the risk of inhaling gastric contents, must be reduced as this may also be associated with loss of vitreous. Neuroleptanalgesia is suggested as a method of inducing anaesthesia but special attention must be paid to the patency, and safety, of the airway. Intubation of the trachea and controlled ventilation are normal practice..

## EAR, NOSE AND THROAT

### Aural surgery

*Special factors*
1. Control of bleeding
2. $N_2O$ diffusion into air spaces
3. Assessment of hearing or vestibular function during anaesthesia
4. Assessment of facial nerve function

1. Use of a vasoconstrictor by the surgeon
   Avoidance of venous congestion by the anaesthetist
   Hypotensive anaesthesia (p 117)
2. A rise in pressure occurs as $N_2O$ diffuses into the middle ear. If a tympanic membrane graft has been inserted it may become dislodged. The administration of nitrous oxide should cease at least 30 min before the graft is applied, and even this may be considered by some to be a conservative estimate. If 100% oxygen is administered following the use of nitrous oxide it is possible to produce a negative pressure within the middle ear cavity. Ventilation with an oxygen/air mixture prevents pressure gradients developing.
3. Intra-operative communication with the patient is usually reserved for those who are undergoing surgery of the ossicles or labyrinthine ablation.
   Isolated forearm   —the application of a tourniquet during the injection and subsequent distribution of non-depolarising muscle relaxants allows the function of a limb to be retained, and on lightening the anaesthetic a response can be elicited from a command.
   Evoked responses—auditory stimulation results in a change in the electrical discharge on the surface of the cerebral cortex, this is termed an 'evoked response' and can be used to test auditory function during anaesthesia. Changes in frequency or amplitude in the EEG response to sound are commonly seen as in the non-specific K response.

4. Avoidance of neuro-muscular blocking agents allow facial movements to be seen should the drill irritate the facial nerve.

## Nasal surgery

*Special factors*
1. Control of bleeding
   Moffett's method—application to the nasal mucosa of 2 ml of 8% cocaine and 2 ml of 1% sodium bicarbonate.
2. Control of diabetes insipidus following transnasal hypophysectomy
   Pitressin tannate injection or pituitary snuff
   Other hormone replacement therapy—thyroxine
   —corticosteroids

## Pharyngeal/laryngeal surgery
Preservation of the airway is the main problem

*Tonsillectomy*
*Guillotine*: premedication—atropine
          anaesthesia—nitrous oxide/oxygen/halothane
          position—supine using Doyen gag
*Dissection*: anaesthesia—intravenous induction agent/nitrous oxide/oxygen/halothane.
          a) Boyle Davis gag to allow per-oral insufflation
          b) Intubation with suxamethonium—Doughty tongue plate modification of Boyle Davis gag
   (Nasal intubation should be avoided in children as the adenoids are often inspected or removed. In adults nasal intubation with a streamlined cuffed tube allows use of controlled ventilation if desired. Spontaneous ventilation is often preferred. A sandbag under the shoulder allows extension of the neck.)

Post tonsillectomy bleeding
1. Large quantities of blood may have been swallowed
2. There may be evidence of severe loss of blood (low blood pressure, rapid pulse, sweating, peripheral cyanosis) apart from the visual evidence in the mouth

Management: order of events
1. Set up blood transfusion
2. Use lateral head down position, clear pharynx of blood clots
3. Administer oxygen
4. Inhalational induction—nitrous oxide, halothane and oxygen
5. Intubate with cuffed tube
6. At end of operation, some authors suggest removing blood from the stomach

*Laryngoscopy*
Laryngeal visualisation —'deep' halothane anaesthesia with
                        spontaneous ventilation
Laryngeal biopsy        —a)  muscle relaxant combined with
                           perlaryngeal insufflation
                        b)  Apnoeic diffusion oxygenation
                           (p 174)
Laryngeal microsurgery—Pollard, Carden or Coplans tube
                        Alternatively, ventilation using a venturi

## DENTAL SURGERY

*Outpatient*—sedation/local anaesthesia and general
             anaesthesia
*Inpatient* —a)  general anaesthesia for dental extractions
            b)  maxillo-facial surgery

### Anaesthesia for outpatient dental surgery

*Contraindications*
1. Full stomach
2. Cardiovascular disease
3. Respiratory disease, both upper and lower respiratory tract
4. Drugs, e.g. hypotensive agents, anticoagulants, β-adrenergic
   blocking drugs, steroids, insulin
5. Endocrine disease, i.e. thyroid disease, diabetes mellitus,
   pituitary disease
6. Miscellaneous; porphyria, 1st trimester of pregnancy, abnormal
   haemoglobinopathies including thalassaemia and sickle cell
   disease or trait

*Indications for general anaesthesia*
1. Infection
2. Failed local anaesthesia
3. Age—young children
4. Allergy to local anaesthetic agents
5. Mental retardation
6. Neurological disease associated with involuntary movement
7. Multiple extractions in different quadrants of the mouth

*Special factors*
Consent
Escort home

*General factors*
Unprepared/incompletely investigated patients
Maintenance of airway
Posture during the procedure
Residual effects of drugs

*Sedation/local anaesthesia*
Sedation/local anaesthetic techniques are particularly applicable to reduce discomfort during prolonged treatment and for patients with dental phobia. The Jorgensen technique involves the intravenous injection of pentobarbitone, pethidine and hyoscine. Another technique uses intravenous diazepam and the injection of a local anaesthetic agent. Diazepam in propylene glycol is irritant to veins and ought therefore to be injected into large veins, however a new formulation in lipid is less irritant.

Patients should be supine during treatment. The glottic reflex may be obtunded and reduced muscle tone may lead to respiratory obstruction. The aim should be to maintain verbal contact with the patient; airway safety is then more assured.

Recovery is delayed after the Jorgensen technique, but less after diazepam. Patients can generally leave the surgery 90 min after injection. They must be accompanied by a responsible adult and must not control machinery or drive a car for at least 24 h. Diazepam may obtund involuntary movements in athetoid patients thereby avoiding the need for general anaesthesia.

Relative analgesia is a technique whereby a 20–30% mixture of nitrous oxide in oxygen is administered via a nasal mask. This maintains verbal contact and facilitates the injection of local anaesthetic in the anxious individual.

*General anaesthesia*
In children an inhalational induction using oxygen, nitrous oxide and halothane is usually routine. In adults however induction may be by intravenous injection using thiopentone (recovery relatively prolonged), methohexitone (initial recovery rapid), propanidid (danger of anaphylactoid reaction) and diazepam (normally used for basal sedation, not suitable for induction of anaesthesia, recovery may be prolonged after a sleep dose).

There has been much discussion concerning the relative demerits of the upright position. On balance the fully horizontal position is probably safest. However, while the horizontal position reduces the danger associated with a severe fall in blood pressure in the upright position, it is more difficult to control the patency of the airway. The airway requires protection from dental debris and this can be attempted by the judicious placement of an oral pack.

Recovery may appear to be rapid; however, approximately 10% of patients feel sleepy the next day. Indeed EEG changes may still be detected even though performance at tests of skill has returned to pre-anaesthetic levels. The patient requires to be escorted home, should not operate or control machinery, or drive a car, take sedatives, tranquillisers, hypnotics or alcohol for at least 24 h. Tests of recovery are generally of little value and certainly do not offer more information than the unsophisticated Romberg test.

**Anaesthesia for inpatient dental anaesthesia**
Many inpatient dental anaesthetics are given to patients whose
medical condition makes them unsuitable for outpatient treatment.
Pregnancy, cardiac disease, anxiety and mental retardation make
up a large proportion of such patients.

*Dangers of nasal intubation*
Nasal intubation is commonly practised for the inpatient, the
airway is secured and, if the endotracheal tube is cuffed or an
adequate oropharyngeal pack used, then the airway is protected.
   Damage to the nasal mucosa with severe haemorrhage may
occur or infected debris may be pushed down the nasal passages
into the larynx. In addition the diameter of the nasal tubes that are
used is less than an equivalent oral tube in the same patient; this
increases the resistance to flow and may be an indication for
mechanical ventilation.
   Other factors of particular interest include the danger of bleeding
in the upper airway and cardiac dysrhythmias due to dental
manipulation. Dysrhythmias are thought to be less in those patients
ventilated using a 'balanced' anaesthetic than in those breathing
spontaneously using a volatile agent.

**Anaesthesia for maxillo-facial surgery**

*Special factors*
Intubation in the presence of possible bleeding and oedema
Wired jaw
Control of emesis
Risk of meningitis related to nasal intubation in those patients with
a fracture of base of skull
   The mandible, maxilla and floor of the mouth may be involved in
the surgery; therefore intubation is required. Intubation should be
performed with the patient breathing spontaneously if it is likely to
be difficult due to anatomical deformity resulting from tumour,
trauma or certain well defined syndromes such as
Treacher – Collins. The choice between nasal and oral intubation
depends on the site of the surgery and possible invasion of the
airway by tumour or oedema, or gross deformity due to trauma.
Prolonged surgery suggests the need for controlled ventilation.
   Recovery presents special problems. If the jaws have been wired
together, airway control may be difficult and vomiting becomes
particularly hazardous. The use of an anti-emetic is advisable. It is
advisable to leave a nasopharyngeal airway *in situ* during recovery
and to have wire cutters available in case severe airway obstruction
occurs.
   Meningitis may follow nasal intubation particularly in those
patients with a fracture of the base of the skull.

## ANAESTHESIA FOR 'GENERAL' SURGERY OF THE HEAD

**Parotid surgery** (nerve stimulator required)
Spontaneous ventilation permits the use of a nerve stimulator
which is required to confirm identification of the Facial nerve.
  Induced hypotension may be required, though venous oozing can
be controlled by a 10° head-up tilt.

**Plastic surgery**
Hypotension may be required, see p 117
  For surgery involving superficial structures a basal sedation/local
anaesthetic technique may be used (diazepam or
neuroleptanalgesia). The patency and safety of the airway is always
of prime importance and the maintenance of verbal contact is
desirable.

## ANAESTHESIA FOR SURGERY OF THE NECK

**Posterior approach**
1. Decompression of cervical cord
2. Stabilisation of diseased/traumatised vertebrae
3. Repair of meningomyelocoele

*Special factors*
Immobility of cervical spine—difficult intubation
Orthopaedic fixation frame enveloping chest and head—difficult
intubation
Danger of cord compression with neck flexion (in rheumatoid) and
neck extension (certain cervical fractures)

*Management*
*If a difficult intubation is anticipated . . .*
— psychotropic/dissociative/tranquilliser type premedication to
  facilitate awake intubation if other methods inappropriate
— A stylet (introducer—a stiff, but malleable, wire) should be
  available and equipment for cricothyroid puncture (see p 30)
— Armoured endotracheal tubes—to avoid kinking
— IPPV—prone position—p 80, 111
— Correct posture—avoiding compression of abdomen (IVC), neck
  veins, eyes and nose

**Anterior approach**
1. Thyroid surgery
2. Tracheotomy
3. Laryngectomy
4. Spinal surgery

## Thyroid surgery

*Problems*
Possible metabolic disturbances
Identify patient at risk by tachycardia, hypotension, atrial fibrillation and heart failure (p 66)
Possible tracheal compression causing intubation difficulties
Tracheomalacia may lead to post-operative tracheal collapse
Tracheal compression by post-operative haemorrhage
Recurrent laryngeal nerve damage may lead to hoarseness or stridor and re-intubation may be necessary. Check vocal cord movement at time of extubation.

*Excision of parathyroids*
In the postoperative period a calcium infusion may be required to maintain blood calcium level and avoid muscle spasms. In calcium deficiency states there is a tendency to laryngeal spasm and increased cardiac irritability leading to ventricular fibrillation.

## Tracheotomy

As an acute immediate procedure see p 122

*Elective tracheotomy*
If the upper airway is a problem then the routine described on p 29 should be followed to ensure safety during the intubation sequence. The entire procedure may be carried out using an 'airway and mask' technique or under local anaesthesia using a regional block (p 127) or by local infiltration.
   Assuming tracheal intubation is possible then surgical exposure of the trachea, and construction of the tracheostome, is followed by careful withdrawal of the endotracheal tube to a point above the opening. A sterile tracheostomy tube is then inserted and connected to a sterile set of respiratory hose compatible with the breathing system in use.

## Laryngectomy

*Problems*
The tumour may encroach on the airway making intubation hazardous or even impossible. Great care should be taken over the induction of anaesthesia should the patency of the larynx be in doubt. A preliminary tracheotomy may be necessary; surgically this is less than satisfactory.
   Loss of airway management by anaesthetist when the surgeons excise larynx. A separate set of sterile respiratory hose should be available.
   Excision of thyroid and parathyroids. See above.

## Spinal surgery

Similar problems may be encountered as those described for the posterior approach to the cervical spine, p 89. Distraction of the cervical spine is usually necessary to enable the insertion of a bone graft to span adjacent vertebrae. The skull calipers provide a traction point.

## SURGERY OF THE CHEST

### Anaesthesia for surgery involving the rib cage
1. Correction of pectus excavatum/carinatum
2. Fixation of flail chest
3. Derangement of rib cage associated with kyphoscoliosis (see next section).

In each condition the integrity of the chest wall is abnormal, surgery may result in an increase in vital capacity and an improvement in cardiac performance may occur. In 2. fixation of the flail segment should improve respiratory function.

*Management*
1. Endotracheal intubation and controlled ventilation to ensure adequate pulmonary ventilation.
2. Post-operative analgesia selected to avoid ventilatory depression.

### Anaesthesia for surgery of the thoracic spine
The rib cage may be disorganised by kyphoscoliosis, it may result from neurofibromatosis, Friederich's ataxia, poliomyelitis, spinal tuberculosis, spinal fracture, spinal neoplasia and Marfan's disease.

Severe spinal curvature reduces both the vital capacity and total lung volume (restrictive disease). The lung volumes are further decreased with increasing spinal curvature (reduced FRC) leading to a reduction in the ventilation perfusion ratio with arterial hypoxaemia and hypercarbia in the presence of a high oxygen consumption.

*Surgery unrelated to an existing kyphoscoliosis* (see page 34)
Pre operative identification of pulmonary and cardiac disease and institution of correct control therapy. Patients may be chronically hypoxaemic and intubation may be extremely difficult. Patients must therefore be preoxygenated and IPPV during anaesthesia will be necessary. IPPV may also be required in the postoperative period.

*Surgery for kyphoscoliosis* (Harrington operation)
The intention is to reduce and to arrest progress of the spinal curvature by vertebal fusion and internal fixation using metal rods. The operation is extensive and there may be severe blood loss during surgery and in the postoperative period. Blood loss may be reduced by using an appropriate posture and by keeping the mean intrathoracic pressure low. On the other hand, although induced arterial hypotension may be helpful, it may exacerbate the bleeding if this is primarily due to venous oozing (congested epidural veins).

The prone position may lead to a rise in intra abdominal pressure, thereby reducing or preventing venous return from the lower limbs, leading to increased blood loss. Communication with the patient during anaesthesia (p 84) may be considered desirable to detect cord damage during traction on the vertebrae.

## Anaesthesia for pulmonary surgery
Pulmonary resection occasionally may lead to right ventricular failure associated with a sudden rise in pulmonary vascular resistance and to a reduction in pulmonary performance leading to respiratory failure.

*General considerations*
1. Careful pre-operative assessment of cardiorespiratory reserve
2. Maintenance of gaseous exchange during surgery on the lungs or main airways.
3. Control of secretions (page 119, 190)
4. Postoperative respiratory complications

*Resection of lung tissue*

Pre-operative assessment
1. Medical history including character, and amount, of sputum and an assessment of dyspnoea.
2. General clinical examination
3. Examination of the range of chest movements and air flow (spirometry)
4. Blood gas analysis (objective assessment of pulmonary function)
5. Capacity for work (examination of exercise tolerance)
6. *Cardiac assessment*—Clinical assessment of right ventricular function and pulmonary hypertension, right ventricular strain (ECG).
   Theoretically the likely effect of resection of diseased lung on pulmonary artery pressures may be determined during cardiac catheterisation by occluding the arterial supply to the diseased lung.

Management
1. Endobronchial intubation and one lung anaesthesia (p 190, 117)
2. Lateral or Parry Brown position (p 111, 112)
3. Assessment of the adequacy of one lung, if there is doubt, by clamping the pulmonary artery to the diseased lung. Reduction of the shunt fraction should lead to a rise in $P_aO_2$.
4. Though digoxin was used routinely during thoracic surgery, it was stopped usually 24–48 h before surgery to obviate the occurrence of dysrhythmias associated with potassium deficiency. Digoxin may be required for the control of ventricular tachycardia, or atrial flutter and fibrillation, and is often administered if the pericardium is opened.
5. After pulmonary surgery a chest drain, sometimes two, is attached to an underwater seal in order to facilitate pulmonary expansion and pleural cavity drainage. Following pneumonectomy care must be taken not to reduce the pressure in the pleural cavity lest cardiac function is compromised by displacement of the mediastinum. If a chest drain is inserted it is clamped off and only released, once an hour, to determine the amount of postoperative haemorrhage.
6. Where possible a policy of extubation with spontaneous ventilation should be followed. This prevents the application of high airway pressure or the tip of the endotracheal tube reopening the sutured, or stapled, bronchial stump.

*Tracheal resection*
Tracheal resection is carried out for either a stricture or a tumour. An inhalational induction should be used to preserve spontaneous ventilation. Intubation with an armoured tube should be performed without the use of a muscle relaxant. A stricture or tumour may permit only a small diameter endotracheal tube to be passed. A muscle relaxant may be used after the airway has been secured. If intubation with an endotracheal tube fails it may be possible to pass a bronchoscope past the narrowing and ventilate using a venturi. During surgery the distal portion of the trachea is intubated once the resection has been performed. The posterior aspect of the trachea is sutured and then the original endotracheal tube is repositioned so that the distal segment is intubated via the proximal segment. The suturing of the anastomosis is then completed. (Cardiopulmonary bypass has been used to facilitate tracheal resection.)

Spontaneous ventilation should be resumed post-operatively to avoid trauma to the tracheal suture line by the endotracheal tube. Excessive coughing during extubation may damage the tracheal suture line.

*Drainage of an empyema*
A history of copious purulent sputum suggests a connection
between an empyema and the tracheobronchial tree. Precautions
must therefore be taken to prevent flooding of the airways with
pus.
  The classical approach is to use local anaesthesia in the sitting
position for rib resection and drainage of the abcess cavity.
General anaesthesia however may be used for rib resection. The
requirements are a smooth induction of anaesthesia with the
empyema in a dependent position. Spontaneous ventilation should
be allowed until the main airways are intubated and separated by a
double lumen tube or a bronchial blocker. The patient may then be
turned so that the empyema is uppermost and IPPV can be
instituted. The abcess cavity is normally drained by a large-bore
tube. Bronchoscopy, using spontaneous ventilation, is indicated if a
bronchopleural fistula is thought to exist and if surgical
intervention is considered.
  *Note*:  The empyema must be dependent
           Spontaneous respiration must be maintained

*Pleurectomy/excision of bullae or cysts*

General considerations
Possible increase in tension in an existing pneumothorax or cyst
Air leak in the postoperative stage

General management
1. If a chest drain is not in situ then facilities for the insertion of a
   chest drain should be immediately available.
2. Endobronchial intubation: IPPV may lead to an increase in
   tension within the pneumothorax or cyst and therefore
   spontaneous ventilation is preferred until isolation of the
   involved lung is assured. Distribution of nitrous oxide within
   all closed gas containing cavities may lead to an increase in the
   volume of gas and therefore the pressure in the pneumothorax
   or pulmonary cysts, and should therefore be avoided.
3. IPPV should be avoided postoperatively to reduce the likelihood
   of an air leak. See section on management of chest drains (see
   page 120).

**Anaesthesia for oesophageal surgery**
1. Transthoracic hiatus hernia repair
2. Oesophageal resection
3. Tracheo-oesophageal fistula

*Transthoracic hiatus hernia repair*

General considerations:
Danger of regurgitation

## Management
Pre-oxygenation followed by cricoid pressure during intubation to prevent regurgitation of gastric contents. Endobronchial intubation is not essential but one lung anaesthesia improves surgical access. A left-side double lumen tube, which is easier to position, is frequently used.

A nasogastric tube is normally inserted; it aids the surgeon during mobilisation of the oesophagus, but may be withdrawn at the end of the operation.

### Oesophageal resection

General considerations
The patient may be in a state of chronic undernutrition.

## Management
Preoperative parenteral nutrition should be considered if the patient is hypoproteinaemic.

Rehydration will be necessary if dysphagia is severe—many litres of colloid and crystalloid may be necessary.

Operative management is the same as that described for hiatus hernia repair with the added problem of more prolonged surgery with its attendant problems of heat and fluid loss.

### Tracheo-oesophageal fistula (TOF)
Tracheo-oesophageal fistulae are usually of the congenital variety although fistulae can occur as a result of neoplasia or prolonged endotracheal intubation. The congenital variety may be associated with cardiac defects.

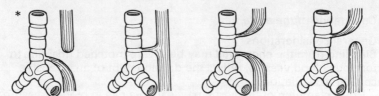

*Most common

**Fig 3.1** Four configurations of tracheo-oesophageal fistula

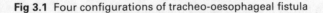

### Management of the neonate with congenital TOF

Preparation
A chest infection associated with contamination of the airway with feed and/or saliva must be treated before surgery. A nasogastric tube of the double lumen Replogle type should be passed to allow

cleansing and emptying of the oesophageal pouch. Hydration should be maintained intravenously. X-ray investigation is required to determine the position of the fistula. (TOF in the neonate is not considered an emergency procedure and the preparation as described above should be carried out).

Anaesthesia
The neonate should intubated, with a single lumen tube, whilst breathing spontaneously.

Ventilatory movements will indicate whether the fistula has been intubated, in which case the tube must be repositioned.

Spontaneous respiration may be maintained until the chest is opened or, alternately, a tentative manual inflation of the lungs may be performed to assess the ability to inflate the lungs and observe whether stomach inflation occur. All other matters pertaining to neonatal anaesthesia must of course be considered, p 15.

Tracheo-oesophageal fistula in the adult should be managed in a similar way to that described for the patient with a bronchopleural leak in that a the double-lumen tube should be used to isolate the lung with the leak. Surgical access is improved and contamination of the lungs with oesophageal contents is limited.

**Anaesthesia for surgery of the great vessels** (not involving cardiopulmonary bypass)
1. Coarctation of the aorta
2. Patent ductus arteriosus
3. Pulmonary artery banding
4. Blalock procedure

*Coarctation of the aorta*

General considerations
Bleeding from the chest wall may be severe (notched ribs, due to tortuous blood vessels, reflect the development of an extensive collateral circulation).

Cross clamping of the aorta may lead to a rise in blood pressure followed by a marked fall when the clamps are removed.

Measure the blood pressure above the below the coarctation. The blood supply below the coarctation is via the collateral circulation and hence the blood pressure below the coarctation is lower than that above.

Though severe hypotension may occur immediately after the clamps are removed, postoperative hypertension may occur and should be treated by sedation and posture. If it is persistant a specific antihypertensive agent may be required.

Management
1. Monitor blood pressure above and below the coarctation (arm and leg)
2. Monitor CVP
3. Induction should be designed to maintain the blood pressure
4. Prepare for massive blood transfusion (p 122)
5. A hypotensive technique may be considered to reduce bleeding
6. Endobronchial intubation with one lung anaesthesia (p 117, 190)

*Patent ductus arteriosus*
During intra-uterine life approximately 80% of the fetal blood ejected into the pulmonary artery is short-circuited into the aorta. During the first 3 weeks of neonatal life the ductus closes permanently. If however the patency of the ductus persists then it is usually surgically close before irreversible pulmonary hypertension occurs (<8 years).

*Pulmonary artery banding*
This is a palliative measure designed to reduce the pulmonary artery blood flow and is used in the management of pulmonary hypertension and in the presence of cardiac septal defects with a left to right shunt.

*Blalock procedure*
This is a palliative measure designed to increase pulmonary artery blood flow in order to increase oxygenation in severe pulmonary stenosis and cyanotic congenital heart disease. Systemic blood is allowed to pass, some for a second time, through the pulmonary circulation by the creation of an artificial fistula between the pulmonary and systemic circulations.

For these latter three procedures the cardiac output and pressures within the separate cardiac compartments and great vessels should be maintained constant to avoid a disruption in the flow pattern with an increase in hypoxia and myocardial strain.

Ketamine increases pulmonary artery pressure and may alter the amount and even the direction of the flow through the shunt, it may therefore be considered unsuitable in these conditions.

In children one-lung anaesthesia is technically difficult and is not therefore usually employed.

**Anaesthesia for surgery involving cardiopulmonary bypass** (CPB)
1. Coronary artery surgery
2. Valve replacement
3. Repair of anatomical defects

Early techniques (Drew) involved the use of hypothermia to temperatures of 10–15°C. During the cooling process two blood pumps are used; one pumps blood from the left atrium through a heat exchanger into the systemic circulation and a second pumps blood from the right atrium into the pulmonary artery for oxygenation in the lungs. The circulation may be stopped as soon as profound hypothermia is achieved. The method suffers from the prolonged preparatory period with the use of two pumps and multiple cannulation.

The general principles used in cardiopulmonary bypass are described below.

1. *Partial CPB*

| | | |
|---|---|---|
| Femoral vein | → | Femoral artery |
| or  Left atrium | → | Aorta |
| and | | |
| Inferior vena cava | → | Pulmonary artery |

The technique of partial cardiopulmonary bypass has been used to enable cooling of the whole body. The partial CPB augments the depressed cardiac output and therefore increases the arterial flow.

(The technique has been used recently to improve oxygenation for patients with severe potentially reversible pulmonary disease (ARDS); the results are not very encouraging.)

2. *Full CPB*

Superior vena cava ⎫ → Oxygenator → Aorta
Inferior vena cava ⎭                    → Coronary arteries

This technique is used routinely for most open heart surgery—coronary artery cannulation is used during surgery of the aortic valve.

3. *Haemodilution*
A priming volume is required for the oxygenator and this must be sufficient to provide a reserve of blood (25% of the minute volume flow) which, in the event of a temporary cessation of venous return to the pump, will be available for the patient, thereby reducing the danger of air being drawn into the circuit and causing an air embolus. The use of whole blood may be associated with coagulation defects and impaired postoperative lung function. Gadboys homologous blood syndrome, which includes functional and histological changes particularly in the lungs, has been linked with the use of large volumes of donor blood.

Crystalloid solutions including Hartmanns solution or 5% dextrose are used in modern haemodilution techniques. Albumen may be added to maintain oncotic pressure. Dilution is limited only by the concomitant reduction in oxygen carrying capacity; on the other hand a reduction in blood viscosity, including that associated with hypothermia, can improve venous return and tissue perfusion.

In adults the dilution should not generally reduce packed cell volume below 30%. Whole blood may be used to prime the oxygenator for use with an infant because the priming volume is much greater than the infant's own blood volume.

### 4. Control of venous return (to the CPB pump)
Normally passive by using gravity. The operating table is set at a fixed height above the inlet to the pump. Active suction may cause collapse of the veins around the cannulae or the ingress of air.

### 5. Oxygenators
a) Rotating disc and screen oxygenators effectively disperse blood in oxygen. They are expensive and require a large priming volume.

   b) Bubble oxygenators allow oxygen bubbles to pass with the blood through a column, thereby giving rise to a froth. Bubble size is an essential consideration. Large bubbles favour carbon dioxide removal whereas small bubbles favour oxygenation. However, small bubbles are not easily eliminated from the blood. The froth bubbles are largely dissipated on a silicone antifoam surface and remaining bubbles are trapped in the settling reservoirs. Disposable bubble oxygenators which require only a small priming volume are available.

   c) Membrane oxygenators. These are unfortunately expensive. They do, however, by using a membrane to interface the blood and oxygen, mimic the normal relations between blood and gas in the lungs. The duration of bypass can be extended using this method. This may be largely due to the preservation of the plasma proteins which may be destroyed by repeated exposure to a large blood-gas interface.

### 6. Control of anticoagulation
Heparin (3 mg. $kg^{-1}$) is given intravenously through a central line, after two hours 1 mg. $kg^{-1}$ is given for one further hour or pro rata. Heparin anticoagulation should be reversed by the use of protamine. Generally speaking 2 mg of protamine will reverse 1 mg of heparin. However the blood heparin may be titrated against protamine standards to determine more accurately the required protamine dose. Sometimes the heparin protamine complex is broken down with resulting prolonged anticoagulation. Loss of fibrinogen may produce a similar effect and should be excluded as a cause of bleeding before giving more protamine.

### 7. Cardioplegia
Cardiac surgery is easier if the heart is still. Cessation of organised myocardial activity can be brought about by inducing ventricular fibrillation by the passage of a low voltage direct current across the

heart, by causing hypoxia by clamping the aorta above the coronary arteries or by perfusing the coronaries with a potassium containing solution. Ischaemic damage to the myocardium can be minimised by bathing the heart in cold saline—care must be taken that local myocardial damage is not caused by ice particles.

### 8. Hypothermia
Cooling is carried out using the pump so that temperature gradients are minimised.

See p 159 for physiology and dangers, eg. quick rewarming—gas embolisation possible

### 9. Gas embolism
See p 80

### 10. 'Cardiac' output
A flow from the bypass pump of less than 2.4 $1.m^{-2}.min^{-1}$ tends to cause metabolic acidosis. 80 $ml.kg^{-1}.min^{-1}$ is a flow calculation that is commonly used. Tissue perfusion is more dependent upon the peripheral resistance than on the absolute flow rate.

### 11. Inotropic agents
See p 154

### 12. Mechanical cardiac support

Intra-aortic balloon counterpulsation
In severe myocardial failure an improvement in coronary perfusion may result in improved myocardial contractility. The purpose of the intra-aortic balloon is to maintain the diastolic pressure so that an increase in coronary artery flow occurs. The device, a balloon that can be inflated with $CO_2$ or He, is positioned in the upper aorta via a femoral artery. It is triggered by the ECG and inflates during diastole; this prevents the egress of blood from the ascending aorta and hence maintains the diastolic pressure. The balloon deflates during systole.

### 13. Postoperative monitoring
Pressures in systemic artery
   central venous system
   wedged pulmonary artery
   left atrium
Cardiac output
Urinary output
Clotting studies
Urea and electrolytes
ECG
Arterial gas tensions
Core and peripheral temperature (a useful guide to survival)

## ABDOMINAL/PELVIC SURGERY

### Abdominal wall (including diaphragm)

*Herniorrhaphy*

Inguinal/femoral
Congenital hernia may be related to a myopathy and rarely this
may carry an increased risk of malignant hyperpyrexia.

Hernia developing later in life may be related to a persistent
cough associated with chronic bronchitis.

Either general anaesthesia or local anaesthesia, epidural, spinal
or local infiltration, may be used. There are no conditions which are
an absolute indication for a particular approach to anaesthesia but
clearly respiratory depression and cardiovascular instability must
be avoided in patients who have myocardial or pulmonary disease.
Infiltration of local anaesthetic agent in the region of the incision
has much to commend it for the poor risk patient.

Omphalocoele, gastroschisis, diaphragmatic hernia, incisional
hernia
All the conditions listed above, in which abdominal organs are
prolapsed outside the peritoneal cavity, are associated with
ventilatory impairment when the extra-abdominal organs are
returned to the repaired abdominal cavity. Omphalocoele may lead
to peritonitis unless surgically closed and this surgery is urgent.
Limitation of pulmonary expansion may lead to hypoxia and
cyanosis. The condition is commonly congenital but may result
from trauma. Positive pressure ventilation is required and surgical
repair is essential.

For the repair of a gastroschisis, congenital diaphragmatic hernia,
or an omphalocoele, muscle relaxation is required and elective
postoperative ventilation should be considered.

### Abdominal vascular surgery

*Aortic surgery*

Hazards      —Ischaemic heart disease and arteriosclerosis
             —Renal artery involvement
             —Friable tissues
             —Maintenance of blood volume (may be impossible
               in the presence of a massive leak)

Management—Preoperative assessment of cardiovascular function
               pp 36–44
             —Induction of anaesthesia without cardiovascular
               depression. (If the aorta is bleeding it is advisable
               not to use neuromuscular blockers. Muscle tone in
               the abdominal wall may maintain the blood
               pressure by preventing further bleeding.) A 'G' suit
               has been found to be useful in maintaining the
               central blood volume.

—Central venous, peripheral venous and arterial cannulation in this situation is required
—Urinary catheterisation is also helpful, urine flow is a good indicator of tissue perfusion
—Anticoagulants are administered as requested
—NaHCO₃ (50 mmol) may be given before the removal of the femoral artery clamps, this compensates for the washout of acid metabolites from the ischaemic legs
—Postoperative IPPV may be required

*Saddle embolectomy*
Hazards        —The patient may be very ill; even moribund
—Patients usually have an arteriopathy and an obvious source of emboli such as valvular heart disease or a recent myocardial infarct
Management—Local anaesthesia unless uncooperative. Blood volume should be maintained and supportive measures taken as required.
—The ECG, CVP and blood loss should be monitored

*Renal artery surgery*
Renal artery surgery is usually required to relieve a stenosis.
Hazards        —Hypertension may be exacerbated by anaesthesia and lead to intracranial haemorrhage however hypotension may occur with myocardial infarction and acute renal failure.
Management—Preoperative assessment and antihypertensive therapy are important, the latter should be continued throughout the period of surgery. Myocardial depression and hypotension should be avoided. Should hypotension occur expand the blood volume. Pressor drugs should be used with great caution and if used select the drug to be effective in the presence of the antihypertensive medication. Ketamine and pancuronium may lead to a marked rise in blood pressure. Monitor the ECG, CVP and blood loss; ensure that the blood volume is maintained.

**Upper abdominal general surgery**
Oesophageal surgery see p 94
Gastric surgery
Gall bladder and hepatic surgery
Splenic surgery
Pancreatic surgery
Small bowel surgery

*General considerations*
Postoperative ileus—nasogastric tube, see p 115
Postoperative pain / respiratory complications, p 144
Electrolyte disturbances may occur due to prolonged vomiting or
diarrhoea. These should be corrected.
Obstruction at the pylorus may lead to reduced gastric emptying
and regurgitation during induction of anaesthesia.
Traction on the vagal fibres in the upper abdomen during
cholecystectomy or vagotomy may lead to bradycardia.
Portal hypertension may lead to haematemesis, with a resulting
acute anaemia; liver failure may co-exist. Porto-caval anastomosis
operations are generally prolonged and usually involve a
trans-thoracic approach.
Excision of the spleen is usually carried out because of trauma,
extreme size or for haematological reasons. If platelets are to be
administered they should be administered after the splenic artery
has been ligated.

*Management*
Anaesthesia is normally induced intravenously. Intubation is
accomplished using a muscle relaxant, suxamethonium (if a rapid
intubation is required) a non-depolariser if regurgitation is unlikely.
Anaesthesia is maintained using inhalational or intravenous agents
combined with full muscle relaxation and IPPV.
   Peripheral venous cannulation is normal practice and
intravenous fluids are given to compensate for pre-operative fluid
deprivation and intra-operative losses. These losses may be great if
the large surface area of the intestine is exposed or handled
excessively. Fluid is lost into the serosa due to the handling
(oedema called the 'third space') and evaporation results in heat
loss as well as fluid loss.

*Liver transplant surgery*
Hazards          —Failure of drug metabolism
                 —Reduced cardiac output after the inferior vena cava
                   is clamped
                 —Sudden rapid loss of blood—massive transfusion
                   p 122
                 —Acidosis resulting from donor liver releasing cold
                   acid perfusate rich in $K^+$. Treatment—$CaCl_2$ +
                   $NaHCO_3$.
                 —Anaemia
                 —Impairment of hepatic function leading to bleeding
                   and reduced plasma cholinesterase. Clotting
                   deficiencies require investigation.
                 —Blood sugar levels should monitored as
                   hypoglycaemia is possible
                 —Hypothermia is a common problem

*Management*—All drug doses should be adjusted p 55
—Owing to gross inequality of ventilation perfusion in some of these patients IPPV may be required postoperatively
—Renal failure due to bacterial toxins may occur and a diuretic may therefore be given prophylactically during surgery
—Facilities for massive transfusion are essential
—Intensive monitoring is mandatory

*Renal surgery*

Nephrectomy/pyeloplasty/pyelolithotomies
*Hazards*        —Position—the lateral position leads to $\dot{V}_A/\dot{Q}_C$ imbalance. Ventilation is biased to the upper lung during IPPV and blood flow to the dependent lung.
—Vena caval compression may reduce venous return leading to a fall in cardiac output
—Renal function disorder, p 50
*Management*—It is important to maintain cardiac output and gas exchange
—If renal failure is not severe general anaesthetic techniques using IPPV may be used provided nephrotoxic drugs are avoided (methoxyflurane)
—Suxamethonium may, in theory, lead to a rise in plasma $K^+$ concentration in uraemic patients
—Both narcotic and volatile agents may be used to maintain anaesthesia, halothane however may lead to hypotension

Renal transplantation
*Hazards*        —This is normally carried out as an urgent procedure and time for preparation of the patient may be limited
(donor kidney ischaemic time when warm—30 min; cold ischaemic time at 4°C – 16 h)
—Chronic renal failure, p 50
(Uraemia/anaemia/hypertension/electrolyte disturbance)
—Haemodialysis, p 164. Hypovolaemia and hypokalaemia are possible if the patient is recently dialysed.
Overhydration and hyperkalaemia if not dialysed.
*Management*—Avoid drugs which may produce hypotension
—Avoid drugs which are not metabolised and are solely excreted by the kidneys (gallamine). Atracurium is a useful muscle relaxant in this situation.

—Blood transfusion should be avoided if possible to avoid inducing antibody formation
—Oxygen delivery to the tissues must be assured—hypoxia is difficult to detect in the very anaemic patient
—Monitor the ECG to identify dysrhythmia, particularly during the induction of anaesthesia, associated with hyperkalaemia
—Avoid the indiscriminate use of veins and avoid any likelihood of damage to the shunt or A–V fistula—haemodialysis may still be required

## Lower abdominal and pelvic surgery
Colectomy
Anterior resection of sigmoid colon
Abdomino-perineal resection
Bladder surgery
Gynaecological procedures

*Hazards*: Postoperative ileus—p 115
    Abdominal incision, pain may affect respiration
    Trendelenberg/Lloyd Davis/Lithotomy positions—p 112
    Deep vein thrombosis—p 119

*Management*: Balanced anaesthesia
    Spinal or epidural anaesthesia, p 128, 130
    Combination of general and local anaesthesia
    Colonic anastomoses—neostigmine—pressure rises within the bowel may cause a leak
    Replacement of blood loss

## Perineal/periperineal/transperineal surgery
Perineal surgery is eminently suited to local anaesthetic techniques, p 128

Circumcision and haemorrhoidectomy are particularly painful procedures and a combination of a local anaesthetic and general anaesthetic technique has been advocated. Postoperative comfort is certainly enhanced by the continuation of the profound analgesia provided by local anaesthetic.

Dilatation of the anal sphincter can cause cardiac dysrhythmias and the pulse should be monitored.

The lithotomy position, together with a request for head-down tilt, may embarrass respiration and for a prolonged procedure tracheal intubation and IPPV should be used.

Anaesthesia should never be induced in the lithotomy position if the patient is likely to regurgitate—the third trimester of pregnancy, hiatus hernia or a recent meal. The patient cannot be turned quickly and the patient's airway is therefore at risk.

## LIMB SURGERY

Operations on the limbs can be divided into three categories, orthopaedics, vascular and superficial minor surgery. For any of these procedures a local anaesthetic technique is possible, the limbs are eminently suited to regional blocks, see p 128.

### Vascular surgery

Vascular surgery of the limbs does not specifically require muscle relaxation thus neuromuscular blockade is not essential, however some microvascular procedures may take many hours and a technique that employs tracheal intubation and IPPV using neuromuscular blockade may be preferred as the recovery period is likely to be less prolonged. For microvascular surgery, which is very dependent on good tissue perfusion for success, a Biers block using guanethidine as the intravenous agent, should be considered as this results in prolonged vasodilatation—a dose of 15 mg of guanethidine diluted with a local anaesthetic solution administered as described on p 138 is adequate. The blood pressure should be monitored as there may be a transient hypertension on release of the tourniquet.

The patient who requires the construction of an arterio-venous fistula will require the preparation and management that is described for patients with chronic renal failure, p 50.

The most common vascular surgery of the legs, stripping, tying or avulsing varicosities, usually requires the patient to be in the Trendelenberg position. Head-down tilt is associated with diaphragmatic splinting and respiratory embarrassment; IPPV should be considered. IPPV is mandatory if the patient is to be prone for ligation of varicosities on the posterior aspect of the legs.

### Orthopaedic surgery

Orthopaedic surgery involving the more distal portions of the limbs can be carried out under 'airway and mask' anaesthesia—the decision to 'intubate and ventilate' being dependent upon the duration of surgery. Surgery on the shoulder or upper arm is more safely, and conveniently, carried out if the patient is intubated as the airway is then secure and the anaesthetist in less proximity to the surgeon.

The problems associated with hip surgery are the problems associated with anaesthesia for the elderly, p 18. The most common hip surgery carried out on the elderly is that of internal fixation of fractures of the neck of femur due to a fall. There is some evidence to suggest that a spinal local anaesthetic technique may reduce postoperative morbidity. Early mobility is desirable.

Methylacrylate cement which is used to secure orthopaedic prostheses to bone can cause hypotension. This hypotension can be limited by preloading of the patient with intravenous fluid. Careful monitoring is essential. Theories as to the cause of the hypotension include excess monomer and gas embolism or fat embolism due to a rise in pressure inside the lumen of the bone shaft. This may be secondary to the insertion of the prosthesis into the shaft and the rise in temperature that results from the chemical reaction that occurs during the setting of the monomer.

## ENDOSCOPIES AND RADIOLOGICAL PROCEDURES

### Endoscopies

*Arthroscopy*
See anaesthesia for limb surgery

*Bronchoscopy*

Hazards:
Hypoxia
Cardiac dysrhythmias
Loss of protective glottic reflex

Management
*Local anaesthesia*: (for the cooperative adult)
   1. Spray the palate, pharynx and back of the tongue with a 4% lignocaine solution. Alternatively the patient may suck an amethocaine lozenge.
   2. The superior laryngeal nerves are blocked by passing gauze soaked in the local anaesthetic over the back of the tongue into the piriform fossae. Special curved forceps (Krause) are used for this purpose.
   3. 2 ml of 4% lignocaine is injected through the cricothyroid membrane at the end of a deep expiration. Alternatively the local anaesthetic may be instilled through the glottis, the pharynx and glottis having been previously anaesthetised.
*General anaesthesia*: A general anaesthetic may involve spontaneous respiration or neuromuscular blockade with IPPV. IPPV with paralysis must only be used if it is considered safe to do so (p 35); a bronchopleural fistula may make IPPV ineffective.

The neonate may be bronchoscoped awake, alternatively a deep anaesthetic maintained with a volatile agent in oxygen is also possible—ether is a good agent for this purpose as separation of the patient from the agent does not result in rapid reversal of the anaesthetic state.

Balanced anaesthesia using a hypnotic, an analgesic and a neuromuscular blocking agent is commonly used. Bronchoscopies are normally short procedures and intermittent suxamethonium, or an infusion, is used to provide a muscle relaxation that allows rapid return of power at completion of the procedure. A rapid recovery of consciousness and the return of protective reflexes must be an essential part of the technique.

IPPV is provided by the use of a venturi system that injects oxygen down the lumen of the bronschoscope and entrains air through the open end. This technique has revolutionised bronschoscopy under general anaesthesia; previous methods, inserting an endotracheal tube into the end of the bronchoscope, apnoeic diffusion oxygenation or the simple insufflation of oxygen down the bronchoscope, all resulted in either hypoxia or hypercarbia.

If a fibreoptic bronchoscope is to be used it can either be passed down a rigid bronchoscope, IPPV with the venturi can be continued, or the patient may be intubated and the bronchoscope passed through an air-tight gasket on the connector to the endotracheal tube—ventilation is maintained by a conventional ventilator.

If a biopsy has been taken the patient should be positioned so that any blood drains away from the 'good' lung and up the trachea.

*Cystoscopy*
*Hazards*:     Repeated anaesthetics—many patients have frequent anaesthetics and consideration should be given to the agents used—it has been suggested that halothane should not be used repeatedly within 6 weeks.
*Management*:  Local anaesthetic techniques are suitable if a general anaesthetic is considered undesirable. Most patients having a cystoscopy will be 'daycase' patients and thus a local regional technique would be innappropriate, the agents used to provide a general anaesthetic should be chosen to produce a quick recovery and minimal after effects. The salient points pertaining to 'daycase' anaesthesia are described under Dental Anaesthesia, p 86.

*Peritoneoscopy* (Laparoscopy)
*Hazards*:     Gaseous distension of the abdomen may lead to a reduced venous return, a fall in cardiac output and limitation of diaphragmatic movements
               Possible gas embolism, p 80
               Regurgitation
*Management*:  Local anaesthesia—many tubal sterilisations are now performed using local anaesthesia and a conscious patient
               General anaesthesia—tracheal intubation and IPPV is mandatory

*Laryngoscopy*
See laryngeal surgery, p 86

*Mediastinoscopy*
*Hazards*:    Possible haemorrhage—a mediastinoscope is
                 inserted behind the sternal notch to pass into the
                 upper mediastinum. The potential for serious
                 haemorrhage exists and blood should be available
                 (cross-matched)
*Management*:  The trachea should be intubated with an armoured
                 endotracheal tube and IPPV should be instituted. A
                 peripheral infusion line should be set up.

*Oesophagoscopy*
*Hazards*:    Rupture of the oesophagus
                 Damage to the teeth or jaw
                 Danger of regurgitation if oesophageal contents are
                 held above a stricture.
*Management*:  Oesophagoscopy with a flexible instrument may be
                 carried out under sedation.
                 General anaesthesia with intubation of the trachea,
                 full muscle relaxation and IPPV is necessary if a
                 rigid oesophagoscope is to be used.
                 Intermittent suxamethonium is commonly used to
                 provide the muscular relaxation.
                 An intravenous infusion for 24 hours is necessary as
                 it is common practice for the patient to be 'nil by
                 mouth' for 24 hours post-endoscopy.

*Ophthalmoscopy*
See ophthalmic surgery p 83

**Radiological procedures**

*Neuroradiology*
The specific problems associated with neurological disease (p 57)
are of obvious importance. The working space is usually cramped
but in addition there are specific problems associated with each
procedure.

Air encephalography (pneumoencephalography)
*Hazards*:    Change of posture during the procedure
                 Expansion of gas volume by nitrous oxide
                 Air embolism
                 Herniation of the medulla
*Management*:  General anaesthesia—an intravenous induction,
                 intubation with a flexometallic tube, and
                 spontaneous ventilation is usually satisfactory.
                 Local anaesthesia may be associated with a
                 persistent headache, nausea, vomiting,
                 sweating and vasomotor collapse.
                 Ketamine has been used as the sole agent in
                 children for this procedure.

Cerebral angiography

*Hazards*:     The development of a haematoma in the neck may displace the trachea leading to partial airway obstruction

Hypertension or hypotension

A respiratory arrest may occur if the intracranial pressure is markedly raised

Contrast medium may be injected sub-intimally in the carotid artery or intrathecally

If the procedure is performed under local anaesthesia a burning sensation on the face and in the retrobulbar region may cause movement with the spoiling of the films

*Management*:  Local anaesthesia with sedation, using a neuroleptanalgesic technique, is possible. Careful assessment of the required narcotic dose is necessary to avoid respiratory depression.

General anaesthesia using nitrous oxide with a muscle relaxant, intubation with a flexometallic tube and IPPV is generally preferred. Hyperventilation reduces the $P_a co_2$ and reduces the circulation to normal brain with little effect on the tumour circulation thus improving the definition of the tumour circulation. On the other hand hyperventilation should be avoided if a subarachnoid haemorrhage is suspected. Spasm of blood vessels may be present and a further reduction in blood flow should be avoided.

Computerised axial tomography (CAT scanning)

*Hazards*:     Monitoring at a distance is required during the procedure

Hypoxia, hypercarbia and drugs which increase intracranial pressure should be avoided

*Management*:  General anaesthesia is only required for examination in small children and in adults who cannot keep still. A 'balanced' anaesthetic technique may be used with IPPV.

Nuclear magnetic resonance imaging (NMR)

*Hazards*:     Electrical equipment attached to the patient may disturb the scanning process and the magnet may induce currents in implanted electronic devices such as a pacemaker.

*Management*:  A photoelectric device may be used to monitor the pulse. General anaesthesia is only required for the patients who cannot keep still, as for CAT scanning. Non magnetic connectors must be used.

Arterial angiography
*Problems*:     Generalised cardiovascular disease, p 36.
*Management*:  For coronary and translumbar aortography a light
                general anaesthetic is required and in the case of
                translumbar aortography IPPV with the patient in
                the prone position but without the chest and pelvic
                supports is necessary.
                The ECG and blood pressure must be monitored
                throughout the procedure.

Cardiac studies
*Hazards*:      Those associated with cardiac disease, p 37, 43
                Increased cardiac excitability during the positioning
                of the catheters
*Management*:  General anaesthesia is not usually required for
                cardiac pressure and blood gas tension studies but
                for those unable to cooperate it may be necessary.
                Sedation . . . various regimens for adults
*General anaesthesia*: The $F_1O_2$ and $P_aCO_2$ must be kept constant to
allow interpretation of the blood gas tension results. Intrathoracic
pressure and cardiac contractility should also be disturbed as little
as possible to avoid reversing a shunt e.g. a left to right shunt may
be reversed if a rise in intrathoracic pressure leads to a rise in
pulmonary artery pressure.
    Both spontaneous respiration and IPPV techniques are used—as
long as a particular technique is used in consistently in one
department a reliable interpretation of the results is possible.

## PROBLEMS AND TECHNIQUES ASSOCIATED WITH ANAESTHESIA

### Effects of posture

*Supine*
Muscle relaxation removes the muscle support for the vertebral
ligaments leading to flattening of the lumbar spine with
postoperative backache. The supine hypotensive syndrome is
associated with patients with an intra-abdominal mass, eg.
pregnancy, p 19.

*Prone*
Anterior/posterior expansion of the chest is reduced and diaphragm
movements are reduced if the patient is not supported off the table
to allow abdominal expansion.

*Lateral*
Gravity reduces the blood flow to the upper lung and during IPPV
pressure of the abdominal contents on the dependent hemisphere
of the diaphragm reduces expansion of the lower lung. Ventilation
and perfusion of the lungs is therefore mismatched.

During spontaneous respiration the dependent diaphragm is elevated, because of the pressure of the abdominal contents, and therefore when it contracts it sweeps out a larger volume than the upper diaphragm. Ventilation and perfusion are more equally matched.

If the chest is opened mediastinal shift may occur with deleterious consequences; flow through the inferior vena cava may be reduced and the cardiac output reduced.

### Lithotomy
There is a marked reduction in the vital capacity. Damage to the hip and vertebral joints is possible particularly if they have limited movement.

### Trendelenburg
This steep head-down position results in diaphragmatic splinting and, in the susceptible patient, regurgitation of gastric contents. The airway and ventilation must be protected. The central blood volume is increased.

### Reverse Trendelenburg
This steep head up tilt decreases the central blood volume due to the pooling of blood in the legs. This posture, on its own or in conjunction with depressant drugs, may cause hypotension. Venous ooze is reduced in the elevated parts of the body.

### Parry Brown
This position has been used to facilitate the drainage of secretions from the tracheobronchial tree during thoracic surgery. The patient lies prone with the hips elevated above the level of the shoulders and the head turned to the side of the operation. The arm on the operative side hangs down by the side of the table. On opening the chest there is no mediastinal shift.

Nerve damage can occur in many positions—excessive abduction of the arms and depression of the shoulders (brachial plexus), outside aspect of lower legs against lithotomy poles (lateral popliteal) and compression of the upper arm (radial nerve).

## Cannulation of vessels

### Peripheral veins

AVOID
Sites in the proximity of joints
Infusions in the legs (increased incidence of thrombophlebitis/thrombosis)
Irritant fluids e.g. urea; a second cannula should be used for such fluids

Change the cannula either 24-hourly or, more realistically, at the first sign of any tissue reaction.

*Central veins*

Routes
*Antecubital fossa*: The antecubital fossa can be used for the insertion of central venous catheters and either the basilic or cephalic vein may be cannulated. The course of the cephalic vein passes through the clavipectoral fascia and it is at this point that the cannula may be held up. the basilic vein passes more deeply, becoming the axillary vein, and passage of the catheter is less likely to be impeded.

An X-ray must be taken to confirm the position of the tip of the catheter.
*Subclavian*: The subclavian vein passes over the first rib and then medially and downwards. Its highest point is just medial to the midpoint of the clavicle.

To cannulate this vessel the patient should be supine with the head turned away from the site of insertion. Head-down tilt is desirable—this fills the vein and minimises the risk of air embolism. The cannula is inserted 1 cm below the lower border of the clavicle and just lateral to its midpoint. It is directed to go below the clavicle and in the direction of the suprasternal notch. On the left side the thoracic duct is a structure that may be damaged.

X-ray confirmation of position is desirable.
*Internal jugular*: At its lower end the internal jugular vein is covered by the sternomastoid muscle.

With the patient supine, head down and with the head turned away from the site of injection the cannula is inserted 3 cm above the clavicle and just lateral to the lateral border of the sternomastoid, the needle being directed towards the supra-sternal notch.

X-ray confirmation of position is desirable.
*External jugular*: The external jugular vein is superficial and crosses the sternomastoid muscle. It is relatively easy to cannulate but it may be difficult to get the cannula to pass into the subclavian vein.
*Femoral*: The femoral vein lies medial to the femoral artery which is found at the midpoint between the anterior superior iliac spine and the public symphysis. It can be cannulated and with a catheter of sufficient length it can be used to record central venous pressures.

Uses
—Measurement of central venous pressure to assess blood volume
—Parenteral nutrition
—Haemodialyis

## Complications

The complications of central venous cannulation include pneumothorax, hydrothorax, haemothorax, cardiac tamponade (due to perforation of the atrial wall by the cannula) and it is also possible to create an arterio-venous fistula.

### Arteries

### Brachial artery

The brachial artery crosses the elbow joint anteriorly. Its anatomy is variable and it can be considered an end artery as its occlusion can result in distal ischaemia if the collateral circulation is insufficient.

It is superficial, being covered only by skin and fascia, and cannulation is not difficult.

### Radial artery

It is found lateral to the tendon of flexor carpi ulnaris at the wrist. Before cannulation of this artery a test should be carried out to establish that there is a patent ulnar artery.

*Allen's test*: The hand is exsanguinated with compression of the radial artery and ulnar artery—subsequent release of the ulnar artery should result in a flushing of the hand if circulation via the ulnar artery is adequate.

### Femoral artery

The femoral artery passes deep to the inguinal ligament, midway between the anterior superior iliac spine and the public symphysis. The vein lies medial and the nerve lateral to the artery.

### Dorsalis pedis

The dorsalis pedis artery is found on the dorsum of the foot between the tendons of extensor hallucis longus and extensor digitorum longus, at the root of the cleft between the first and second toes.

A modified Allen's test should be performed on the foot with occlusion of the dorsalis pedis and the posterior tibial arteries.

The general technique for cannulation of arteries is:
1. Test for adequacy of collateral circulation
2. Palpate and fix artery by skin tension or by straddling the artery with fingers
3. Either enter the artery directly or transfix it with the needle or cannula
4. If transfixed then the cannula is withdrawn into the lumen and then advanced

Uses
—Pressure monitoring
—Blood sampling
—Cardiac output measurement
—Haemodialysis

Complications
Ischaemia in the distal tissues supplied by the artery
Haemorrhage
Nerve damage if artery and nerve adjacent

### Choice of $P_a\text{CO}_2$ during anaesthesia
To hyperventilate or not? That is the question.

*Hypocapnia*
Sympathetic tone is less
Cardiac output is decreased
There is a lesser degree of vasodilatation
The pain threshold is raised thus MAC values are decreased
resulting in a reduction of drug dosage
Postoperative respiratory depression is possible due to the
hypocapnia

*Normocapnia*
Sympathetic tone is not reduced as in a state of hypocapnia
Cardiac output is maintained—cardiac irritability may be increased
Postoperative depression due to hypocapnia is impossible
Greater doses of drugs are required to maintain the patient pain
free and the muscles relaxed
To ventilate, or not ventilate?
   The answer to this question depends on several factors.
1. Airway resistance.
     Nasal endotracheal tubes > oral endotracheal tubes
     Double lumen tubes > single lumen tubes
2. Need for muscle relaxation by the surgeon
3. Need to control the $P_a\text{CO}_2$
4. Need to intubate
5. Duration of operation

### Naso-gastric intubation
Nasogastric intubation is carried out
—to facilitate aspiration of gastric secretions
—to detect and monitor gastric and small bowel stasis—
   for feeding.
   Nasogastric intubation should only be carried out if it is
necessary as it has certain disadvantages that can be of a serious
nature.

It increases the incidence of chest infections, destroys the integrity of the cardiac sphincter, irritates the pharynx, and mal-positioning may result in instillation of fluids into the lungs with potentially fatal results.

For details of naso-gastric feeding regimen see p 168.

## Pulmonary aspiration syndrome

The inhalation of gastric contents is associated with a large proportion of 'avoidable' anaesthetic deaths.

Its occurrence in obstetric anaesthetic practice is termed Mendelson's syndrome and has a high mortality rate although when it was originally described (1946) it did not. Some factor(s) involved in modern anaesthetic or obstetric practice may be altering the picture of the condition.

The effects of acid in the lungs include inflammation, exudation and the production of haemorrhagic oedema fluid. Hyaline membranes occur and there is destruction of lung parenchyma. The pH of the acid has to be below 2.5 to produce this picture in experimental animals.

Factors which increase the risk of regurgitation should always be noted and attempts made to minimise the risk. Active emptying of the stomach either by the passage of a stomach tube or by the use of an emetic is possible and the positioning of the patient another. Head-up tilt, if the situation allows, will prevent passive movement of gastric contents up the oesophagus and thence into the airway.

The prophylactic use of antacids is now routine in obstetric anaesthesia and is described on p 20.

Protection of the airway by endotracheal intubation is mandatory if the patient is at risk and the rapid intubation sequence, with cricoid pressure, should be followed, p 79.

Management of the pulmonary aspiration syndrome

1. The airway should be cleared of gross contaminants by head down tilt and suction. Bronchoscopy may be necessary. Oxygenation should be maintained and intubation is desirable.
2. Bronchial lavage is then carried out in an attempt to reduce further chemical irritation by the inhaled acidic fluid. 0.9% saline is probably the least hazardous solution to instil—alkaline solutions have been used in an attempt to neutralise the acid but are irritant themselves.
3. Steroids are given for their anti-inflammatory effect; bronchospasm may also be reduced
4. Specific agents may be required for the treatment of bronchospasm—e.g. adrenaline, aminophyline, salbutamol and atropine
5. Respiratory failure may ensue and IPPV should be instituted. The general problems are dealt with on p 156.

**One lung anaesthesia**
One lung anaesthesia may inadvertently be used if a single lumen endotracheal tube slips down the right main bronchus. Following intubation chest movements and air entry should be checked to ensure that this situation does not exist or persist.

One lung anaesthesia is electively used during intrathoracic procedures where the inflated lung would impede surgical access or where there is a large air leak from one lung making effective ventilation difficult. Many endobronchial tubes have been designed for the purpose (p 190) but the most common double lumen endobronchial tube in use today is the Robertshaw—it is designed so that it is easy to position and the internal cross sectional area is maximised thus reducing the resistance to ventilation and making the passage of a suction catheter for aspiration of secretions easier.

The effects of ventilating one lung and collapsing the other are variable in degree from one patient to another.

The greatest physiological change occurs in those patients with normal lungs as the passage of a large proportion of the cardiac output through an unventilated lung results in systemic hypoxia. The patient who has had an occluded main bronchus for some time, due to neoplasia, will show little change.

Shunts of between 20% and 65% of the cardiac output may result from the passage of blood through the unventilated lung 20 minutes after deflation of the lung. Hypoxia can be minimised by increasing the inspired concentration of oxygen—this maximises the oxygenation of blood passing through the ventilated lung. If high concentrations of oxygen are used care must be taken to ensure that the patient is unaware of the proceedings.

Tidal volume and frequency of ventilation may need adjusting to maintain alveolar ventilation but at the same time keeping the airway pressure minimal. Venous return to the heart is reduced due to the exposure of the mediastinal veins to atmospheric pressure. If mediastinal shift occurs, and the great veins become kinked, then a catastrophic fall in cardiac output may result.

On reinflation of the lung all segments must be checked to ensure full aeration. Atelectasis of the underlying lung can be a problem—some workers have used positive end-expiratory pressure to minimise it.

**Induced hypotension during anaesthesia**
A good surgical field may be produced by the use of a tourniquet on an exsanguinated limb, by the use of local vasoconstrictor agents or by the use of induced hypotension.

The major hazard of induced hypotension is cerebral ischaemia and thus the indication for hypotension is the virtual impossibility of surgery without a bloodless field. The benefits must outweigh the risks.

Certain patients are more obviously at risk, those with a past history of cerebral ischaemia and those with an existing oxygen transport problem.

*General principles*
1. Continuous cardiovascular monitoring is essential and cerebral function monitoring is ideal as it is impossible to predict the adequacy of cerebral perfusion in advance. IPPV is usually employed during induced hypotension as the physiological dead space may be 80% of the tidal volume, however, spontaneous respiration is used by some as a means of monitoring medullary perfusion.
2. The practice of good general anaesthetic techniques minimises the need for specific hypotensive agents.
—No venous congestion due to respiratory obstruction or coughing
—Reduced sympathetic tone by adequate oxygenation, ventilation and analgesia
3. Posture—the use of a physical method to produce a degree of hypotension is a great safety factor in that it can be reversed quickly if necessary. The monitoring of blood pressure must take into account the pressure difference between the site of measurement and the brain due to the weight of the column of blood in the vessels.
4. Drugs that produce depression of the myocardium and vasculature, such as halothane, are commonly employed. A reduction in cardiac output, however, is not desirable.
5. Ganglionic blockade, either by specific agents or by agents that have this action as a side-effect, is also used. Halothane, d-tubocurare and spinal and epidural anaesthesia fall into the latter group, hexamethonium, pentolinium and trimetaphan into the former.
6. Sodium nitroprusside has specific action on vascular smooth muscle and when administered as an infusion produces a controllable fall in peripheral resistance, arterial blood pressure and central venous pressure. Heart rate and cardiac output rise. Care must be taken not to administer a toxic dose in either total amount given or in the rate at which a lesser dose is given. The antidote, sodium nitrite and vitamin $B_{12a}$, must be available.
7. If a compensatory tachycardia negates the effect of the hypotensive agent being used then a $\beta_2$ adrenergic receptor blocker may be used—other causes for a tachycardia should be excluded.

Many techniques are used to induce hypotension during anaesthesia, the ability to reverse this unnatural state, quickly if necessary, should be built into the method.

Under normal circumstances the blood pressure should be allowed to rise slowly, haemostasis should be secured and blood loss should be replaced.

Good postoperative care with pain relief and oxygen by mask are essential as restlessness and hypoxia may result in reactionary haemorrhage or organ ischaemia.

**Control of intravenous drug concentrations**
The physicochemical properties of a drug, the degree of protein binding, the regional distribution of blood flow and in some instances active transport mechanisms determine to which of the variety of 'compartments', within the body, the drug is distributed.

The volume of distribution, a purely mathematical concept, is expressed as

$$V_D = \frac{X}{C}$$

where X = total amount of drug
C = plasma concentration

Drug distribution may be confined to anatomical compartments; for example, heparin is confined to the plasma water.

To the extent that the volume of distribution affects drug concentration it also influences drug action. If the pharmokinetics of a particular drug's distribution are known, the administration may be planned to maintain a near constant circulatory concentration. Multicompartmental computer models have been constructed to improve the control of drug administration and hence the predictability of their effects.

In clinical practice a loading dose of the drug is usually given followed by a constant infusion if rapid achievement of the desired concentration/effect is necessary. The infusion rate is then adjusted according to the patient's response.

**Respiratory physiotherapy**
Breathing exercises in the preoperative period may be used to increase the vital capacity by encouraging diaphragmatic movements and effective coughing.

Postural drainage of both diseased segments and apparently normal areas of the lungs allows secretions to collect in the main bronchi. These may then be cleared by coughing.

For those patients who require IPPV pulmonary physiotherapy, application of vibratory movements to the chest wall, postural drainage and associated pulmonary expansion by squeezing of a reservoir bag has proved effective in maintaining good pulmonary ventilation and preventing atelectasis.

**Deep vein thrombosis prophylaxis**
Deep vein thrombosis frequently occurs in the veins of the calf, though other parts of the peripheral venous system may also be involved. Immobility during prolonged surgery or during the

postoperative period may lead to venous stasis which may, particularly when associated with dehydration and altered blood coagulability, progress to deep vein thrombosis.

Diagnosis may be made on clinical evidence, i.e. swollen ankles and tenderness in the calf, but is confirmed using either the Doppler ultrasound technique or the uptake of $^{125}$I-labelled fibrinogen. Though swollen ankles may be inconvenient, the serious hazard is pulmonary embolism associated with severe chest pain, dyspnoea and right ventricular failure.

Venous stasis may be reduced by hydration and the use of physiotherapy, elastic stockings, leg elevation and intermittent compression of the calf muscles by pneumatic leggings. In high-risk patients the prophylactic measures must be continued throughout the period of risk, that is until the patient is ambulant. High-risk patients are those who have a past history of venous thromboembolism and those patients undergoing abdominal or pelvic surgery for malignant disease. One third of these patients may develop a deep vein thrombosis; 2% may suffer a fatal pulmonary embolus. Many other factors predispose to thrombus formation: age, obesity, varicose veins and infection; early postoperative mobility is essential.

External pneumatic compression of the calves may be used in conjunction with any of the other prophylactic measures.

The prophylactic use of low dose heparin, oral anticoagulation and Dextran have been shown to be of value.

5000 units of heparin 2 hours preoperatively and 8-hourly postoperative is effective but this regimen has a slightly increased risk of wound haematoma; a 12-hourly postoperative regimen does not.

Oral anticoagulation, which doubles the prothrombin time, reduces thrombus formation but increases the risk of bleeding to an unacceptable level. A lesser degree of anticoagulation reduces this risk but does not prevent thrombi forming although it may reduce thromboembolism.

Dextran 70, 500 ml at the time of operation and daily for up to 5 days, is effective prophylaxis. There is a slight risk of bleeding but it may also cause overloading of the circulation in those patients with incipient cardiac failure.

**Chest drains**
The function of a chest drain is to allow gas or fluid to leave the pleural space at the same time preventing the ingress of air.

There are two commonly-used sites for the insertion of chest drains: the anterior thoracic wall in the second intercostal space and in the mid-axillary line in the 5th or 6th intercostal spaces. The latter is preferable as it is more comfortable for the patient and the resulting scar is in a less noticeable position. Damage to vessels and nerves is avoided if the trocar is inserted immediately above the lower rib, as the nerves and vessels lie under the inferior border of the ribs. Large intrathoracic vessels are unlikely to be damaged if the 1–2 cm of intercostal space just lateral to the sternum is avoided.

Following a pneumonectomy a chest drain may be inserted to allow assessment of postoperative bleeding. It is normally clamped off and only released intermittently to assess the loss. In this situation the chest drain may also be used to adjust the position of the mediastinum if a shift has occurred—air may be allowed into the space or removed from it as the situation dictates.

Following a lobectomy, or similar procedure where lung tissue remains in the hemithorax, the chest drains are used to evacuate the pleural space of air which encourages the inflation of the lung. They may be connected to a low pressure vacuum pump for this purpose ($-5$ to $-10$ cmH$_2$O).

If the chest drain has been inserted as a treatment for a tension pneumothorax then it should under no circumstances be clamped or attached to a vacuum pump. The flow of gas through the chest drain may exceed the capacity of the pump and thus the pump will retard the drainage of the gas and a tension pneumothorax may re-occur.

## Defibrillation

Defibrillation is the passage of an electrical current across the heart to terminate ventricular fibrillation (VF) or to convert atrial and ventricular tachyarrhythmias (VT) to normal rhythm.

*Ventricular fibrillation*

7000 V for a few thousandths of a second stops the chaotic electrical activity and, by synchronising the refractory periods of the muscle fibres, allows the pacemaker to regain control.

*Ventricular tachycardia*

Depolarisation of the whole heart during the refractory period allows the sino-atrial node to regain control.

Direct current defibrillators can deliver up to 400 W s in less than 10 ms. Large diameter 'paddle' electrodes are used to prevent burns.

During VF the shock can be given at any time as there is no organised activity; however, a synchronised shock has to be given during cardioversion or VF may result from the electrical pulse coinciding with a T wave—the vulnerable period during the electromechanical cycle. The R wave is used to trigger the defibrillator.

The maximum energy (400 W s (joules)) is used when treating VF, but when a cardioversion is being carried out, a lower level of energy is used (25 W s) and this is increased as necessary.

Electrode jelly must not be allowed to run between the paddles and personnel must keep clear of metal work and water during the administration of the shock.

*Note*: AC defibrillators are not used because they cannot be used for cardioversion (VF is more likely), the convulsion is greater than with DC and the heart rate, blood pressure and contractility are less affected by a DC shock.

## Massive blood transfusion

The transfusion of large quantities of blood (15+ litres) is associated with a high mortality rate. Many of the problems can be anticipated and corrective measures taken.

1. Cross-matching of the blood will minimise the probability of a transfusion reaction.
2. Filtering of blood will remove much of the debris that accumulates in stored blood and will prevent the lungs from becoming loaded with this particulate matter.
3. Warming the blood will reduce the likelihood of hypothermia secondary to the infusion of litres of fluid at 4°C. The temperature of the heating device should not exceed 42°C.
4. A dilutional coagulopathy should be anticipated and a clotting screen should be obtained early in the procedure. If it is normal it will act as a baseline for later results. Platelets and fresh frozen plasma may be required.
5. The potassium and calcium equilibrium may be disturbed but there is little evidence that active measures are required. Citrate toxicity is unlikely unless the metabolic state of the patient is severely impaired—liver failure, hypothermia and renal failure.
6. Stored blood is acidic (pH 6.6–6.7) and there is some rationale in administering alkali to counteract this; blood-gas analysis should be carried out and the acid/base state corrected. In the longer term the citrate will be metabolised and result in a metabolic alkalosis.
7. The problems that are encountered in all transfusions are accentuated when the volumes to be infused are increased—air embolism, infection, transmission of disease and circulatory embarrassment.

Anticipation of the above problems and an accurate assessment of the blood-loss, together with careful monitoring of the circulatory state, should result in a patient who has an adequate circulatory volume, an adequate state of perfusion and adequate oxygen transport.

## Laryngotomy

The advantages of laryngotomy over tracheotomy are that it is very quick, it does not open up tissues in the neck, it avoids dangerous structure and the wound heals very quickly with little scarring.

The head is extended, without rotation, and the cricothyroid membrane is identified. A transverse incision is made and the cricothyroid membrane incised. Intubation of the trachea is then carried out with a tube of appropriate size.

*Note*: A tracheotomy is carried out by extending the head, without rotation, and making a midline incision. The large vessels in the neck are pushed back, with the fingers, behind the sternomastoid muscles. Retraction of the thyroid isthmus upwards enables palpation of the trachea—two or three tracheal rings are incised, 2nd, 3rd or 4th, and the sides of the incision are held apart until a tube is inserted. A stitch may be placed on each side of the incision to hold the sides apart on future occasions. Incision of the first ring may lead to tracheal stenosis, and an incision that is too low may endanger the innominate vessels.

**Australia-antigen (HBsAg) precautions**
Accidental infection with the virus of serum hepatitis can result in serious liver damage or death.

High risk-patients are those who are known to be positive on testing for the Australia antigen, or its antibody, those patients requiring regular haemodialysis, drug addicts and those jaundiced patients in which a diagnosis has yet to be made.
Anaesthesia orientated precautions
To prevent the contamination of skin, eyes, nose and mouth it is suggested that all personnel should be gowned, masked and goggles should be worn.

Venepuncture should be carried out with disposable equipment and the hands should be protected with disposable gloves.

Spilt blood or body fluids should be diluted with strong hypochlorite solution and wiped with a disposable cloth.

All disposable items should be placed in a plastic bag which is sealed and marked indicating its 'high-risk' category.

# 4. Local anaesthetic techniques, postoperative analgesia and the management of chronic pain

## LOCAL ANAESTHETIC TECHNIQUES

### General approach
1. Explain to the patient the nature of the procedure
2. Examine the patient for
   Sepsis
   CNS/Spinal disorders
   Skeletal abnormalities/surface landmarks
   Evidence of a bleeding diathesis or anticoagulant therapy
3. Exclude allergy and anticoagulant therapy
4. Check resuscitation equipment
5. Insert intravenous cannula
6. Position patient
   Prepare site(s) of injection
   Check equipment, needles, catheters, ampoules etc
   Perform block
7. Observe patient for any untoward effects, drowsiness, tinnitus and numbness of lips and tongue, indicative of toxic concentrations of local anaesthetic. Late signs of toxicity are tremors and convulsions.
   (It should be noted that true allergy to local anaesthetic agents is extremely rare and that the signs of CNS toxicity are usually, incorrectly, described as allergy).

## NERVE BLOCKS FOR SURGERY OF THE HEAD AND NECK

### Scalp and cranium
A band of infiltration from glabella, above ear, to occiput blocks all nerves. Inject three layers—skin, subcutaneous tissue and periosteum if bone is to be removed. The temporalis muscle may need to be infiltrated.

## Eye
1. Infitration of eyelids
2. Retrobulbar injection within muscle cone
   (ciliary nerve and ganglion are blocked)
3. Block facial nerve at neck of mandible, just below the zygoma
   (prevents squeezing of the eyeball by orbicularis oculi)

The retrobulbar block may be performed by a superior approach (Macintosh) through the superior rectus with the patient looking down, or by the infero lateral approach (Atkinson) from a point at the inferolateral margin of the orbit passing backwards along the floor of the orbit.

## Nose
Parts of both the I and II divisions of the trigeminal nerve (V) innervate the nose.

Ophthalmic N (I) { Supratrochlear branch of Frontal
                  { Anterior ethmoidal branch of Nasociliary

Maxillary N (II) { Infra-orbital branch
                 { Long sphenopalatine (sphenopalatine ganglion)

Frontal nerve: 1 cm above caruncle; proceed laterally to roof of orbit.
Anterior ethmoidal nerve: Inject 1 cm above caruncle, 3.5 cm along wall of orbit.
Infraorbital branch: Inject 1 cm below orbital margin, directly below pupil.
Sphenopalatine ganglion: Inject 0.5 cm below midpoint of zygoma, anterior to the coronoid. At a depth of 4 cm the lateral pterygoid plate is encountered; advance 1 cm anteriorly into the pterygo-maxillary fissure. Withdraw plunger before injection as the orbit or pharynx may be entered.

## Throat
A tonsil block involves the lesser palatine branch of the maxillary nerve (II division of V) and the lingual branch of the mandibular nerve (III division of V). A glossopharyngeal nerve (IX) block is also necessary.
Technique A local anaesthetic lozenge is sucked and later the upper parts of the anterior and posterior pillars, and the infra- and supratonsillar areas are infiltrated.

The larynx and pharynx

| | | | |
|---|---|---|---|
| *Sensory* | Mucous membrane above cords and below epiglottis | VAGUS N | Internal laryngeal N |
| | Mucous membrane below cords | VAGUS N | Recurrent laryngeal N |
| | Oropharynx, posterior 1/3 tongue | | |
| | Superior surface of epiglottis | GLOSSOPHARYNGEAL N | |
| | Nasopharynx | SPHENOPALATINE N | |
| *Motor* | Cricothyroid, inferior constrictor | VAGUS N | External laryngeal N |
| | Intrinsic muscles of larynx | VAGUS N | Recurrent laryngeal N |
| | Pharynx and palate | VAGUS N | Pharyngeal plexus |

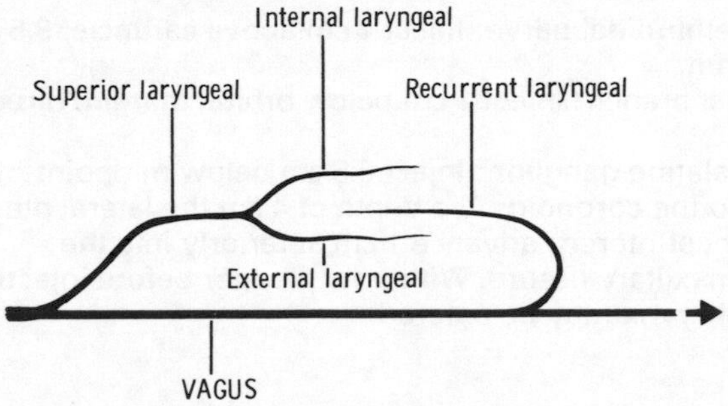

**Fig 4.1** The laryngeal nerves

Vagus nerve block—technique

The patient lies supine and looks straight ahead. The pinna is held forward. A needle is inserted just anterior to the tip of the mastoid process, angled 30° anteriorly. At a depth of 4 cm an aspiration test is carried out and then 2 ml of local anaesthetic is injected, the needle is withdrawn 0.5 cm and a further injection made.

Veins, arteries and nasopharynx may all be punctured and the superior cervical sympathetic ganglion, glossopharyngeal, accessory and hypoglossal nerves may all be affected. Airway obstruction can result.

**Mandibular nerve blocks for dental surgery**
The mandibular nerve is division III of the Vth cranial nerve.
1. Extra-oral approach
The mouth is opened wide and the position of the condyle marked,
the needle is inserted at this point, horizontally and slightly
anteriorly. At 4 cm the lateral pterygoid plate is encountered.
Position a marker 0.5 cm from the skin and redirect the needle
posteriorly. Inject 2 ml of local anaesthetic and 5 ml more as the
needle is withdrawn.
2. Intra-oral approach
Using the index finger, placed lateral to the lower molars, palpate
the anterior edge of the ramus of the mandible. Rotate the finger
into the retromolar fossa and advance the finger to touch the
internal oblique ridge. The needle is inserted 0.1–1 cm medial to
the midline of the fingernail and lateral to the pterygomandibular
ligament. 0.5 ml of local anaesthetic is injected as soon as the
buccinator is pierced (lingual and long buccal nerves are blocked),
advance the needle a further 2.5 cm and inject a further 2 ml. This
will block the inferior dental nerve.

**Cervical plexus blocks for surgery of the neck (Fig 4.2)**
Nerves C2, C3 and C4 lie in the groove between the anterior and
posterior tubercles of the transverse processes of the respective
cervical vertebrae and therefore lie in the plane which exists
between the muscles originating from these tubercles. The
transverse process of C3 lies behind the carotid artery at the level

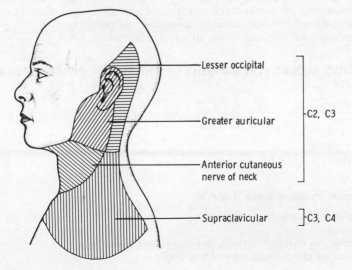

Lesser occipital

Greater auricular

Anterior cutaneous
nerve of neck

Supraclavicular

C2, C3

C3, C4

**Fig 4.2** Sensory dermatomes served by C2, C3, C4

of the hyoid bone. With the patient looking slightly to the opposite side the carotid sheath is displaced medially and a needle inserted to just pass through the edge of sternocleidomastoid, backwards and medially until bone is reached. The needle should be passed beyond the transverse process so that infiltration is ensured on withdrawal. 5 ml of local anaesthetics is injected. C2 and C4 are blocked through the same point of entry through the skin. The phrenic and vagus nerves and sympathetic chain may all be involved.

### Sympathetic blockade

Stellate ganglion
Vascular insufficiency of the upper limbs, pulmonary embolism, status asthmaticus and angina are a few of the indications that have been suggested as indications for a stellate ganglion block.

Paratracheal approach (Moore)
With the patient lying supine the head is extended without a pillow and the needle is inserted 3 cm lateral to, and above, the jugular notch. Advance the needle posteriorly; when the transverse process of C7 is touched, withdraw 0.5 cm and inject 10 ml of local anaesthetic.

Sweating, salivation and bronchial secretions are reduced by the block. Vasodilation occurs and cardiac pain is abolished. Horner's syndrome results, miosis, enophthalmos and ptosis; and the intraocular pressure falls.

Complications are numerous—the phrenic nerve and brachial plexus may be blocked and intrathecal and epidural injections may also be made. Pneumothorax, oesophageal puncture and intravascular injection have all been reported.

### NERVE BLOCKS FOR SURGERY OF THE TRUNK, PERINEUM AND LEGS

Epidural ⎫
Spinal ⎬ Anatomy and physiology—see pp 145–147
Paravertebral ⎭
Intercostal
Autonomic blocks

### Spinal epidural block (Fig 4.3)

*Contraindications*
Sepsis
Problems of haemostasis, anticoagulant therapy
Acute or chronic disease of the CNS

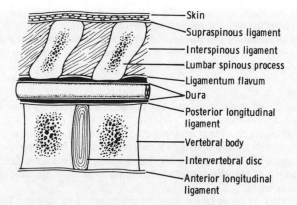

Fig 4.3 Sagittal section through the lumbar spine

| Complications | Treatment |
|---|---|
| Hypotension | —fluids, posture, vasopressor |
| Patchy analgesia | —a larger volume of injectate may overcome the inadequate block |
| Spinal subarachnoid puncture | —see below |
| Epidural abcess or haematoma | —surgical decompression |
| Spinal artery thrombosis | |
| Spinal cord or nerve root damage | |
| Aseptic or septic meningitis | |

*Lumbar epidural*
Technique: The patient is placed in the lateral position with the hips, knees and neck flexed. The back must be perpendicular to the floor and the lumbar spine parallel to the edge of the bed.

Identify the space to be used and infiltrate subcutaneously and then more deeply into the interspinous space. Perforate the skin with a large-bore needle. Insert and advance the epidural needle until the epidural space is located. Confirmation of the needle position may be achieved by either a loss of resistance technique or by a change in electrical conductivity that occurs on entering the space.

Loss of resistance:
Syringe with air or saline
Macintosh balloon
Odom's indicator
Hanging drop method

Local anaesthetic is injected (10–20 ml), if a 'single shot' technique is to be used, or a catheter is inserted 2–3 cm beyond the tip of the needle, the needle withdrawn, a bacterial filter attached and then the local anaesthetic injected.

During pregnancy the spread of the local anaesthetic is increased and only ⅔ of the normal dose is required. In the elderly a reduced dose is also desirable.

Problems
Identification of the space—obesity, calcification of ligaments
Dural puncture—loss of CSF—perform the epidural in another space and inject the local anaesthetic. Physiological saline is infused into the space through a catheter for 24 hours to minimise the leakage of CSF by raising the intraepidural pressure. General hydration must also be maintained. 'Low pressure' headaches may last up to a week.

Blood patches have been used in an attempt to seal the hole; however, their use must be weighed against the possible danger of providing a nidus for infection.
Blood stained tap—try another space up or down

*Thoracic epidural*
A thoracic epidural has similar contraindications, complications and difficulties to that of a lumbar epidural. In addition the vertebral spines are closer together and angled caudally. A lateral approach may be easier that the conventional mid line approach as used in the lumbar region.

Insert a needle 1 cm laterally to the caudal end of the spinous process and infiltrate to the vertebral arch. The epidural needle is inserted and advanced in the same direction but allowed to pass above the arch into the interlaminar space. Further advancement of the needle is made whilst testing for loss of resistance.

The lateral technique is less dependent on spinal flexion, avoids calcified ligaments and allows easy passage of the epidural catheter.

**Spinal subarachnoid block**
*Contraindications*—as for epidural
*Position*—lateral or sitting
*Technique*—a fine-bore needle (25 G) is passed through a guide (a Sise introducer) or a larger standard needle and advanced until CSF is seen in the lumen.

The spread of local anaesthetic is controlled by specific gravity, posture (degree of head up or head down tilt), spinal curvature, the volume and rate of the injection and barbotage. Hypo and isobaric solutions are not now used because of the dangers of a high spinal. The site of action of drug injected at L3, the highest point of the lumbar curve, can be affected by posture.

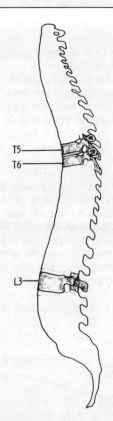

**Fig 4.4** Spinal curves indicating highest and lowest points when the patient is supine

T5–6 is the lowest point of the thoracic curve and local anaesthetic 'pooled' here can be used to provide a spinal anaesthetic for upper abdominal surgery. At this level the block will also interrupt the sympathetic supply to the viscera.

Doses  —1.4 ml  TII
         —1.6 ml  T9
         —2.0 ml  T5

The lumbar region is used for spinal anaesthesia because there is less possibility of damage to the spinal cord, which ends in the adult at the L1/2 level. For 'mid' and 'low' spinals the sitting position is favoured because flexion is more easily obtained, CSF pressure is higher and the dorsal midline is not distorted by sagging skin.

*Complications*
Dry tap
Bloodstained tap—if the CSF remains bloodstained the procedure
may have to be abandoned
Hypotension—posture, fluids, and possibly ephedrine
Total spinal—maintain ventilation and treat hypotension as above
Headache—the smaller the needle the less likely it is that low
pressure headaches will occur; they should be treated
symptomatically and by maintaining hydration. The rapid infusion
of crystalloid solution, 500 ml, can reduce headche.

**Paravertebral block**
The paravertebral space is wedge-shaped. It communicates
laterally with the intercostal space and medially with the epidural
space. It is limited anteriorly by the parietal pleura and posteriorly
by the costotransverse ligament.

Thoracic—weals are raised 3 cm from the midline opposite the
lower borders of the spines. The needle is inserted perpendicular to
the skin until the transverse process is hit. It is then directed over
the upper border of the transverse process and 5–10 ml of the local
anaesthetic is injected.

Lumbar—the weals are raised opposite the upper border of the
spines.

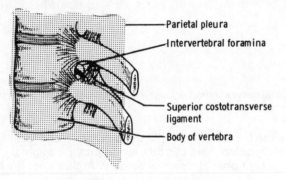

**Fig 4.5** The paravertebral space

**Intercostal nerve blocks**

| Spinal level | Region of anaesthesia |
| --- | --- |
| T2–T6 | from sternal angle to xiphisternum |
| T7–T9 | from xiphisternum to umbilicus |
| T10 | umbilicus |
| T11–L1 | from umbilicus to pubis |

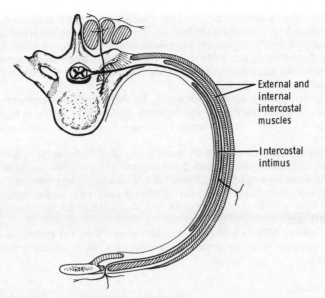

External and
internal
intercostal
muscles

Intercostal
intimus

**Fig 4.6** The course of the intercostal nerves

*Approaches*
1.  At the angle of the ribs
2.  Posterior axillary line
   1.  The angle of the ribs is located at the lateral margin of the
erector spinae muscles. The patient is placed in the lateral position
and two lines are drawn 7–8 cm from the midline, from scapulae to
iliac crests. A needle is inserted at points where the ribs cross the
lines and is then advanced until contact is made with the rib. It is
then withdrawn slightly and redirected below the lower edge of the
rib. 2–3 ml of local anaesthetic is injected.
   2.  The posterior axillary line approach is similar to that described
above except that the posterior axillary line is the longitudinal
surface marking. Using this approach the lateral cutaneous nerves
are not included within the block.

**Autonomic blocks**
Thoracic
Lumbar
Coeliac plexus
   1.  Thoracic sympathetic blockade may be indicated for biliary
and renal colic, acute pancreatitis, angina or asthma. The ganglia
lie on the heads of the ribs covered by costal pleura.

Weals are raised 3 cm from the midline over the transverse processes of the desired vertebrae. The needles are inserted so as to impinge on the transverse process and then slipped inferior to them. A marker is set at 4 cm and the needle advanced in a medial direction. An aspiration test is carried out and 5 ml of local anaesthetic is injected.

2. Lumbar sympathetic block may be indicated in peripheral arterial disease, traumatic vasospasm and acute arterial occlusion. The ganglia lie on the anterolateral aspects of the lumbar vertebral bodies.

Mandl's posterior approach is carried out in the lateral position with the spine flexed. Weals 5 cm lateral to the upper borders of the spinous processes of L2, L3 and L4 are raised. Insert needle perpendicularly for 4–5 cm on to the transverse process and then direct upwards and inwards 3–4 cm. Aspirate and then inject local anaesthetic.

3. Coeliac plexus block is normally performed for the relief of pain originating in the upper abdomen as a result of malignant disease.

*Technique*

Kappis' method
Identify the first lumbar spine and raise a weal 7–8 cm lateral to it—below the 12th rib. Insert a long needle at an angle of 45° to the median plane and in a slightly upward direction and contact should be made with the body of L1. Redirect slightly laterally and glance past the body, advance the needle 1 cm more, aspirate and inject 20–40 ml of local anaesthetic. Hypotension is controlled, if necessary, by infusion of fluid or by a vasopressor.

## SPECIFIC NERVE BLOCKS FOR PERINEAL SURGERY

Saddle Block
Caudal
Pudendal
Paracervical

**Saddle block**
The spread of a spinal subarachnoid anaesthetic block may be restricted by dose and posture such that only the saddle area is affected. A hyperbaric local anaesthetic solution is used in the sitting position.

**Caudal block**
A caudal block is a form of epidural anaesthesia. Local anaesthetic is injected into the epidural space via the sacral hiatus—to block T10–T12 a large volume is required. Dural puncture is rare, as the

dural sac ends at S2/S3. However, the anatomy of the sacral hiatus is quite variable.

Technique: the patient assumes a semi-prone, or prone, position and the sacral hiatus is located between the sacral promontories. A weal is raised and then the needle (large- or fine-bore) is inserted perpendicularly through the sacrococcygeal membrane and advanced until contact is made with the posterior aspect of the sacral body. Withdraw slightly and deflect the hub of the needle into the natal cleft, advance 1 – 2 cm and test for position (aspiration and loss of resistance to air). Local anaesthetic is injected (10 – 20 ml).

Hazards additional to those of lumbar epidural:
1. Possible increased risk of infection
2. Danger of injury to fetus if carried out during the second stage of labour

**Pudendal**

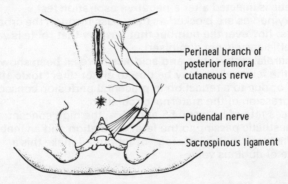

**Fig 4.7** The courses of the pudendal and perineal nerves

S2, S3 and S4 join to form the pudendal nerve 0.5 – 1.0 cm proximal to the ischial spine. It then passes posteriorly to the spines between the sacrospinous and sacrotuberous ligaments. That is, it passes from the greater sciatic notch to the lesser sciatic notch. 50% of inferior haemorrhoidal nerves arise directly from the sacral plexus, and they perforate the sacrospinous ligament and lie close to the tip of the ischial spine.

Transperineal approach: With the patient in the lithotomy position a skin weal is made ⅔ of the way from the anus to the ischial tuberosity. The ischial spine is palpated from within the vagina and a 10 cm needle is directed through the weal to a point just inferior to the spine. 10 ml of local anaesthetic is injected after an aspiration test.

Transvaginal approach: A sheathed needle is held between the first and second fingers and advanced into the vagina until the ischial spine and sacrospinous ligament are palpated by the second finger. The needle is inserted 1 cm at a point 1 cm medial to the spine and 1 cm below the lower edge of the ligament. 10 ml of local anaesthetic is injected.

The perineal branch of the posterior femoral cutaneous nerve is blocked at the latero-posterior aspect of the ischial tuberosity (5 ml) and the episiotomy line should be infiltrated (5 ml).

This is a poor method for producing pain-relief in labour. High concentrations of local anaesthetic cause relaxation of the pelvic diaphragm which reduces the mother's ability to assist expulsion of the fetus.

**Paracervical**
A sheathed needle is inserted into the right and left fornices of the vagina, the needle is then advanced 1–2 cm and 5–10 ml of local anaesthetic is injected after a negative aspiration test.

Sensory nerves are blocked as they pass through the broad ligaments; however the number that pass by that route is variable. Uterine efficiency is not diminised.

Bradycardia, tachycardia and acidosis have all been shown to occur in the fetus which may be due to either direct toxic effects in the fetus or due to a reduction in placental perfusion consequent upon depression of the maternal circulation.

A success rate of between 55 and 85%, the high concentrations of local anaesthetic passing to the fetal circulation and an inability to initiate the block in the 2nd stage of labour all make this a technique of dubious value.


## NERVE BLOCKS FOR SURGERY ON THE LIMBS

*Arm*:  Brachial plexus block
       Circumferential blocks
       Intravenous block
*Leg*:  Lumbar plexus block
       Sacral plexus block
       Circumferential block
       Intravenous block

**Brachial plexus block**

*1. Interscalene technique*
Position the patient supine with the head turned away. A finger is placed behind the sternocleidomastoid muscle, at the level of the 6th cervical vertebra, resting on the anterior scalene muscle. The interscalene groove is located at the lateral edge of this muscle. A needle is inserted into this groove, perpendicular to the skin, and

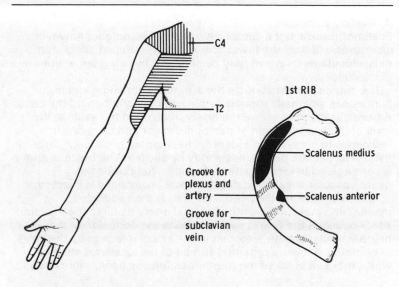

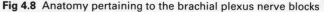

**Fig 4.8** Anatomy pertaining to the brachial plexus nerve blocks

advanced until paraesthesiae are elicited. Aspirate, and inject local anaesthetic if satisfactory. Pneumothorax is not a complication.

### 2. Supraclavicular technique
There are many techniques, but care must be taken to avoid pneumothorax. The 'parascalene technique' (Vongvises and Panijnyanond) is a recently-described method.

The patient lies supine, with the head turned away from the side to be treated, and with the arms by the side. A finger is placed immediately lateral to the sternocleidomastoid, immediately above the clavicle. It will lie on scalenus anterior which is moved laterally. A needle is inserted 3 cm in an antero-posterior direction, 2 cm above the clavical and immediately lateral to the anterior scalene muscle. When paraesthesia is elicited, aspirate, then inject local anaesthetic if satisfactory. If the needle strikes bone (the first rib) without paraesthesia—inject local anaesthetic in a fan-like manner.

### 3. Infraclavicular technique
An advantage with this technique is that the intercosto-brachial nerve (T2) is blocked (Fig 4.8).

The patient lies supine with the head turned away from the side that is to be blocked. A needle is inserted 2.5 cm below the mid-point of the clavicle and advanced laterally towards the brachial artery. Use of a peripheral nerve stimulator may aid confirmation of the correct position.

### 4. Axillary technique

Pneumothorax is not a complication of this technique; however anaesthesia of only the lower arm may be produced. Block of the musculocutaneous nerve may be achieved by using larger volumes of injectate.

The supine patient abducts the arm to a right angle and the humerus is externally rotated by placing the hand behind the head. A needle is inserted above the artery, high up in the axilla at the level of the lower margin of pectoralis major and a change in resistance to pressure will identify the moment of passage through the fascial sheath, paraesthesia may be elicited. The brachial artery is compressed below the site of the inject to occlude the neuro-vascular sheath distally, and local anaesthetic is injected.

After withdrawing the needle the arm is then adducted, maintaining pressure over the brachial artery distal to the injection site. Adducting the arm is said to release the occlusion of the neuro-vascular sheath proximal to the site of injection by the head of humerus, allowing proximal spread of the local anaesthetic, which makes a block of the musculocutaneous nerve more likely.

### Circumferential blocks

Circumferential blocks may be achieved at the elbow and wrist. Subcutaneous and intradermal infiltration is carried out, and depots of local anaesthetic injected to block the median, radial and ulnar nerves in the appropriate positions.

### Intravenous block (Bier)

Technique: insert a cannula into a vein on the dorsum of the hand—a needle is more likely to pierce the vein during the subsequent manoeuvres. A double-cuff tourniquet is positioned on the upper arm. The arm may now be elevated, or an Esmarch bandage applied. If the latter, premedication or some form of analgesia may be necessary. Inflate the proximal cuff on the tourniquet above systolic blood pressure. The local anaesthetic solution without adrenaline is injected—up to a volume of 40 ml of 0.5% lignocaine, for a fit 70 kg man, for an arm—and the solution is massaged into peripheral areas, as the finger tips often retain sensation.

The distal cuff is inflated, and the proximal cuff deflated, strictly in that order. This protects the patient against leak of the local anaesthetic into the systemic circulation, and reduces the pain associated with the tourniquet as the pressure is now applied over an area that has been subject to the action of the local anaesthetic.

If a bloodless field is required the tourniquet is left on; otherwise it may be deflated gradually after the drug is fixed in the tissues, between 5 and 10 minutes.

It is possible for local anaesthetic to seep past the tourniquet through venous channels in bone.

## Lumbar plexus
Iliohypogastric
Ilioinguinal
Genitofemoral
Lateral cutaneous nerve of thigh
Obturator
Femoral

These nerves pass between the quadratus lumborum and psoas muscles, and an extension of their investing fascial sheath may be used to direct the local anaesthetic agent to block the whole plexus, the 'inguinal paravascular technique' (Winnie).

A needle is inserted lateral to the femoral artery and when paraesthesia is elicited in the distribution of the femoral nerve the local anaesthetic is injected. The drug will pass up the fascial cleft and block the lumbar plexus. (Alternative techniques involve multiple blocks.)

## Sacral plexus
Sciatic nerve
Posterior cutaneous nerve
Pudendal nerve

The sciatic and posterior cutaneous nerve of thigh leave the pelvis close together and blocking the sciatic nerve results in a block of the latter also. Only the pudendal then remains to be blocked.

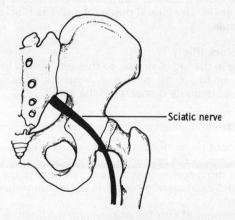

Sciatic nerve

**Fig 4.9** The course of the sciatic nerve in the region of the hip

Techniques for sciatic nerve block

*Posterior (Labat) technique*
A needle is inserted 5– 7.5 cm deep at a point 3 cm below the midpoint of a line joining the posterior iliac spine and the greater trochanter. 10– 15 ml of local anaesthetic is injected.

*Anterior (Beck) technique*
A line is drawn from the greater trochanter parallel to the inguinal ligament. From a point two thirds along the inguinal ligament from the anterior superior iliac spine another line is drawn perpendicular to the first. At this point a needle is inserted to pass on the medial side of the femur. 20– 30 ml of local anaesthetic is injected.

*Lateral (Ichiyanagy) technique*
The patient lies supine with a pillow below the knee. A line is drawn along the shaft of the femur to pass through the posterior border of the greater trochanter. 2 cm beyond the trochanter a needle is inserted 10– 15 cm in the horizontal plane. Paraesthesia should be elicited.
*Note:* Both the lumbar and sacral plexus may be blocked by a lumbar paravertebral approach: see page 132.

**Circumferential blocks**
A circumferential block may be achieved at the ankle. Infiltrate both subcutaneous and intradermal tissues. Depots of local anaesthetic are injected to block the sural, saphenous and medial popliteal nerves at the ankle. The lateral popliteal nerve is blocked near the neck of the fibula.

**Intravenous block** (Bier)
The technique in the leg is similar to that performed in the arm. A large volume, up to 100 ml, of local anaesthetic solution should be used to ensure adequate dispersal of the agent.

**CHRONIC PAIN**

Pain, which could be inadequately defined as the sensation normally experienced in response to a noxious stimulus, is the symptom that most commonly takes the patient to the doctor. Pain of a chronic and excruciating nature is both demoralising and incapacitating.
    The management of chronic pain requires a flexible, multidisciplinary approach and skills in psychotherapy, neurology and local analgesic techniques may be required.
    Pain is a subjective experience and a complaint of pain should never be attributed to imagination or 'nerves'. Exhaustive investigation may eventually uncover an organic basis for the pain.
1. Analgesics
2. Adjuvants

3. Local anaesthetics
4. Steroids
5. Transcutaneous electrical nerve stimulation (TENS)
6. Chemical neurolysis
7. Percutaneous electrical neurolysis
8. Acupuncture
9. Hypnosis

1. Analgesics should be chosen so that the desired pain relief is achieved with minimal adverse effects. Some possible adverse effects, however, may be acceptable in the patient with a terminal condition which would not be acceptable to the patient with a benign lesion.

| BENIGN CHRONIC PAIN | PAINFUL TERMINAL CONDITIONS |
|---|---|
| Analgesia without sedation | Analgesia ± sedation and euphoria |
| Analgesia without addiction | |
| Oral preparation | Addiction not an absolute |
| Avoidance of emesis and constipation | contraindication |
| | Oral, i.m. or i.v. |
| | Control emesis and constipation, if necessary, with adjuvant agents |

Analgesics should be taken at regular intervals so that pain does not return. Taking painkillers 'as required' is usually ineffective.

2. Antidepressants and/or tranquillisers are the mainstay of adjuvant therapy.

Chlorpromazine is often commonly used for its potentiating effect on analgesics, together with its antiemetic and sedative action. In those patients with terminal conditions anti-depressant therapy almost always decreases the analgesic requirements. There is some evidence that plasma serotonin levels are low in patients with persistent pain in terminal illness and that the inclusion of l-tryptophan in the diet counteracts this deficiency and reduces analgesic requirements.

3. The injection of local anaesthetics into painful areas, or to block the somatic nerves serving those areas, may have a duration of effect far greater than that due to its pharmacokinetic properties. One hypothesis is that a vicious circle of pain—muscle spasm—pain may be broken by the single injection and thus produce permanent relief.

4. Steroid preparations may be mixed with local anaesthetic to infiltrate painful sites. Their anti-inflammatory property abates the cause of the pain. Epidural local anaesthesia/steroid mixtures have been used for pain associated with vertebral disc lesions.

5. Chemical neurolysis is used to produce a permanent or prolonged block of pain pathways. 5% phenol in glycerine and 50% alcohol in water are the two commonly used agents. 5% phenol

destroys C fibres and preserves the larger A fibres. Alcohol is painful on injection and can cause persistent pain by causing a neuritis. It is used for sympathetic blocks and for pituitary ablation.

### a. Somatic nerve blocks
When using neurolytic agents on somatic nerves the motor function of the nerve to be blocked must be considered; a block of C2 and T2 to T12, has little adverse outcome. The pain fibres (C) are however, more susceptible to neurolysis than the motor (A) fibres as they are smaller in diameter and unmyelinated.

### b. Sympathetic blocks
Sympathetic tone may be reduced by appropriate blocks and thus help pain caused by excessive sympathetic tone; in addition C fibres travel with the sympathetic nerves.

Conditions for which an appropriate sympathetic block may be helpful:
1. Sympathetic reflex dystrophy
   Causalgia—pain, hyperaesthesia, vasospasm
   Thalamic pain
   Phantom limb pain
   Shoulder–hand syndrome
   Sudek's atrophy
   Post-frostbite syndrome
   Post-traumatic pain syndrome
   Post-traumatic oedema
2. Vascular disorders
   Raynaud's disease
   Thrombophlebitis
   Emboli
   Vasospasm
   Intermittent claudication
3. Pain associated with carcinoma of the stomach, lung, gall bladder, spleen or pancreas (coeliac plexus block)

### c. Subarachnoid blocks
The subarachnoid injection of neurolytic agents can, with care, produce an effect confined to the dorsal nerve root and thus avoid motor effects; the patient must be kept tilted to the appropriate side for 1 hour after the injection. When C3–T1 and L1–S3 are involved possible damage to nerve function and sphincter control must be weighed against the advantages to be gained. 2% chlorocresol or 5% phenol, in glycerine, are used for subarachnoid injection; they are hyperbaric solutions.

### d. Pituitary ablation
Pituitary ablation has been found to relieve pain completely in 40% of patients with disseminated metastatic pain. 1 ml of absolute

alcohol is injected through a transphenoidal needle into the pituitary gland.

6. TENS Transcutaneous electrical nerve stimulation produces pain relief by applying the 'gate' theory of pain to the clinical situation. The theory suggests that stimulation of the large sensory A fibres prevents impulses in the C fibres being transmitted up the dorsal column; that is, the gate is closed. Electrical current is applied through pads strapped to the skin and has been found to be useful in a variety of chronic pain situations.

7. Percutaneous electrical neurolysis/cordotomy.

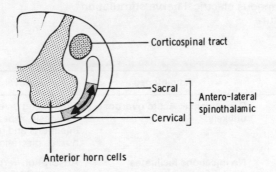

**Fig 4.10** Transverse section through the spinal cord

Radio-frequency-generated heat lesions in the antero-lateral spinothalamic tract can produce pain relief on the contralateral side below the level of the lesion. A needle is passed between the first and second cervical vertebrae, and advanced to penetrate the anterior lateral aspect of the cord. Small stimulating electric currents aid the positioning of the needle before the heat lesion is produced. Cryo-probes are now being used to create lesions, the very low temperatures (−60°C) are achieved by the sudden expansion of gas under pressure—adiabatic expansion. The future application of the technique has not yet been fully explored.

8. Acupuncture is a Chinese method of pain relief that is brought about by 'twiddling' of, or electrical stimulation of, fine needles positioned in the skin at specific locations.

It is thought that the needles may cause the release of endogenous opiate-like substances and some workers have found it of use in the management of persistent pain. Not all members of the population respond to acupuncture.

9. Hypnosis in the responsive patient may provide an alternative method of pain relief. However, it has been found that the analgesic effect may not so readily be achieved after 6 months or so. Patients can be trained to initiate hypnosis on themselves.

## POSTOPERATIVE ANALGESIA

### Methods in common use
Intramuscular injection of analgesics
Oral analgesics
Local anaesthetic and local (epidural) opiate techniques

### Other methods
Cryo-analgesia
Intravenous analgesics
Nitrous oxide inhalation
Transcutaneous electrical nerve stimulation
Acupuncture
Hypnosis

Table 2

| Method | Advantages | Disadvantages |
| --- | --- | --- |
| I.M. | Convenience. Acute overdose unlikely. | Fluctuating levels of analgesia, repeated injections and given at the nurses discretion. |
| ORAL | No injections facilitates discharge home (day cases) | Absorption variable. Not of use if G.I.T. involved in surgery. Fluctuating analgesia. |
| L.A/ EPIDURAL OPIATES | Almost continuous analgesia possible. Profound analgesia allows coughing | All complications associated with L.A. Medically qualified practitioner required for 'top ups'. Possible hypotension and loss of motor power with L.A. and late respiratory depression with opiates. |
| CRYO-ANALGESIA | Reduces use of drugs | Restricted to post thoracotomy pain However, thoracotomy pain is of diverse origins and pain relief is thus incomplete. |
| I.V. | Titration of dosage against pain possible. Continuous analgesia demand systems are available. | Acute overdosage a possibility. Expensive equipment is required, per patient, for demand analgesia. Care and attention of intravenous line necessary. |

| NITROUS OXIDE | Continuous analgesia. Pulmonary performance improved. Use for changes of dressings | Pollution. Danger of bone marrow depression after 48 hours continuous use. |
|---|---|---|
| TENS | Avoids depressant drugs | Controlled trials impossible but its efficacy is not high. |
| ACUP/ HYPNOSIS | Avoids depressant drugs | Time consuming. Low efficacy. |

Pain is a subjective experience and influenced by many factors not easily measured.

### Some general comments

1. Morphine is the standard analgesic with which others are compared
2. A large proportion of patients get as much relief from a placebo as from morphine
3. Increasing the dose of an agent may not necessarily increase analgesia, but the side-effects are increased
4. It is better to give analgesics before pain returns
5. General discomfort accentuates pain
6. Good general analgesia does not protect the patient from pain associated with coughing or physiotherapy
7. Some patients experience greater pain than others
   Neurotics > extroverts
   Central operations > peripheral operations
8. The use of local anaesthetic techniques to provide postoperative analgesia does not markedly enhance respiratory function, as might be expected, although coughing and physiotherapy are not so agonising (intercostal block is possibly superior to epidural block as there is no hypotension or urinary retention that sometimes complicates epidurals—however pneumothorax is a risk)
9. Logistics usually determines the method of pain control used

## ANATOMY OF SPINE, EPIDURAL SPACE AND SPINAL CORD

33 Vertebra—7 cervical, 12 thoracic, 5 lumbar, 5 sacral, 4 coccygeal.

*Vertebrae*
Body
Vertebral arch
Pedicles—grooved to form the intervertebral foraminae
Laminae
Transverse and spinal processes
Articular facets

*Cervical* —1.2.7. atypical—vertebral foramen—artery, vein and sympathetic nerves.

*Thoracic* —1.2.3.4. spines horizontal to oblique
5.6.7.8. spines almost vertical    } Articular facets for ribs
9.10.11.12. oblique to horizontal

*Lumbar* —1.2.3.4.5. No rib facets, no vertebral foramen. Body taller in front than behind; heavy spines horizontal.

*Ligaments*
Anterior longitudinal ligament—axis to sacrum
Posterior longitudinal ligament—axis to sacrum
Ligamentum flavum—Yellow elastic fibres from the articular facets to spinal processes and from the anterior inferior aspect of lamina above to the posterior superior aspect of lamina below.
There is a mid-line cleft between ligamenta flava
Inter-spinous ligament—this connects the spinous processes from root to tip, fusing with the ligamenta flava
Supra-spinous ligament—a continuation of the ligamentum nuchae C7 to sacrum

*Intervertebral discs*
They comprise a quarter of the length of the spine, act as shock absorbers and are made up of the annulus fibrosus and nucleus pulposus.

*Spinal cord and coverings*
Medulla oblongata to L1/2 (neonate L3)
Cauda equina
Filum terminale interna—thread-like extension or cord, ends with dura and arachnoid at S2—continues as filum terminale externa which blends with the periosteum of the coccyx
Dura mater
Arachnoid
Pia mater
   The dura mater is composed of periosteal and investing layers, the latter covers the spinal cord and the former lines the spinal canal. The potential space between the two layers is called the extradual, epidural or, perhaps more correctly, the interdural space.

**Epidural space**
Foramen magnum is the upper limit of the space and the sacral hiatus is the lower. Dural cuffs cover the spinal nerves which pass through the intervertebral foraminae into the paravertebral space. The epidural space is greatest at mid-thoracic level (6 mm).

There are both anterior and posterior venous plexuses and these connect with the intervertebral veins; together they form venous rings at the level of each vertebra.

Branches from the vertebral, ascending cervical, deep cervical, intercostal, lumbar and ilio-lumbar arteries also enter the intervertebral foramina and anastomose in the lateral aspects of the epidural space.

The epidural space is also occupied by fat tissue.

## PHYSIOLOGICAL EFFECTS OF SPINAL/EPIDURAL BLOCKADE

### Nerve conduction

Pre-ganglionic sympathetic fibres are blocked first.

In increasing order of fibre diameter the sensory modalities are blocked; temperature, pain, touch, pressure, and then the motor fibres are blocked followed by the proprioceptor pathways.

### Vascular

Loss of sympathetic tone
Venous pooling due to lack of skeletal muscle tone
Fall in central venous pressure, cardiac output falls
Blood pressure falls

### Respiratory

Spinal – cephalic spread of local anaesthetic may block intercostal nerves or, if higher, the phrenic nerves and cause apnoea
Epidural – respiratory paralysis very unlikely but pain relief more likely to improve ventilation

### Gastro-intestinal tract

The bowel contracts and the sphincters relax. Nausea and retching may still occur.

# 5. Intensive care

## MANAGEMENT OF SEVERE HEAD INJURIES

1. Assessment
2. General supportive measures
3. Specific therapy
   a) to control intracranial pressure
   b) to limit/reduce brain damage
4. Monitoring

### 1. Assessment

*Neurological status*

a) Assessment of conscious level
The level of consciousness is assessed by scoring the responses of
the eye to stimulation and by the responses of the patient to verbal
commands and painful stimuli.
Response to verbal command
   Normal movement to command
   Orientation—self, place, time
   Conversation—confused or innappropriate
   Moans
   No response
Response to painful stimuli
   Purposeful response by limb
   Flexor response—upper limb—rapid withdrawal with adduction
   of shoulder
   Extensor response—forearm pronation, abduction of shoulder
   No response
   (Painful stimuli must not be applied indiscriminately, as pain
   increases intracranial pressure.)
Eye responses
   Spontaneous eye opening suggesting a normal sleep/wake
   rhythm
   Eyes open in response to speech
   Eyes open in response to pain
   Eyes do not open in response to pain

b) Pupil size and reactivity

c) Decerebrate muscle contractions and convulsions

d) Tone / reflexes / abnormal posturing—decerebrate rigidity

e) Thermal homeostasis

f) Cardiovascular / respiratory status
For full assessment see pp 150–161
(Good oxygenation is essential: hypoxia increases the morbidity of a head injury)

## 2. General supportive measures

a) Maintenance of airway
   posture
   oropharyngeal airway $\left. \right\}$ Avoid coughing and straining
   oral endotracheal tube

b) Maintenance of ventilation if necessary. The $F_1O_2$ may require adjusting if the $P_aO_2$ falls. Patients with head injuries are prone to pulmonary oedema.

c) The blood pressure must be maintained but overhydration avoided

d) Control of restlessness / convulsions. Althesin administered by infusion may be valuable as return to the patient's unsedated state occurs rapidly once the infusion is stopped, allowing reassessment within a short time. IPPV using muscle relaxants may be used but full reversal of the relaxant may be difficult to achieve quickly.

e) Feeding should be instituted after the initial assessment period of 24 hours (see p 168). Again, avoid overhydration as the blood/brain barrier is damaged and cerebral oedema occurs easily.

## 3. Specific therapy

a) *Control of intracranial pressure*

 (i) Withholding of fluids will tend to decrease intracranial pressure.

 (ii) Osmotic dehydrating agents may be used to 'buy' time prior to surgery. They are not a definitive treatment as the rebound phenomenon, which occurs after a variable period of time depending on the agent used, will cause an increase in intracranial pressure. Also, leakage of the agent into a haematoma may increase its size.

 (iii) Steroids—usually dexamethasone—are used to reduce cerebral oedema; their mode action is not clear but it is thought that they maintain the integrity of the sodium pump.

 (iv) Intermittent positive pressure ventilation is used to lower the $P_aCO_2$, which in turn reduces intracranial pressure. A $P_aCO_2$

below 3.5 kPa may increase cerebral hypoxia because of the severe cerebral vasoconstriction.

Damaged brain tissue does not respond to changes in carbon dioxide tension and thus will tend to remain well perfused ('luxury' perfusion) when the $P_a\text{co}_2$ is low. If the $P_a\text{co}_2$ is high the reverse occurs and the normal brain 'steals' blood flow from the damaged area which cannot respond by vasodilation ('steal' phenomenon).
(v) Surgical relief of the raised intracranial pressure

b. *To limit or reduce further damage*
 (i) Hypothermia may be of use if the patient is hyperthermic but the overall results are not encouraging; the number of survivors increase, though frequently in a vegetative state.
(ii) Barbiturates—it has been shown in animals that large doses of barbiturates may protect, to some extent, the brain against hypoxic damage. The dose required may depress the cardiovascular system and its place in the traumatised patient is, as yet, to be established.

**4. Monitoring**
Routine monitoring of cardiovascular/respiratory function
Temperature measurement
Fluid balance
Neurosurgical assessment charts
    a) Response to verbal command
    b) Response to painful stimuli
    c) Response of eyes to command or pain
Intracranial pressure monitoring using transducers. Occasionally, due to severe chest wall or intra-abdominal trauma it is necessary to combine IPPV with the use of muscle relaxants. Under these circumstances it is impossible to assess intracranial pressure by the usual clinical means. The intracranial pressure may then be measured directly by placing cannula either in the extra-dural, subdural or intraventricular space. The latter method suffering from technical difficulty including failure to identify the space which may be displaced or obliterated by the raised intracranial pressure. Subdural and intraventricular techniques share the possibility of introducing infection. Extradural techniques, while losing a degree of sensitivity, reduce the incidence of infection.

**FAILURE OF PERFUSION (circulatory failure)**

**Diagnosis**
CVS—Hypotension, tachycardia
CNS—Confusion → unconciousness
Renal—Oliguria → anuria
Temperature—Cold periphery, core temperature raised

## Causes
Relative or absolute hypovolaemia
Pump failure—right- or left-sided or both
These functional causes may result from many processes, each requiring specific treatment.
Trauma—severe haemorrhage external or internal (fractures), loss of plasma (burns)
Bacteraemia—Gram negative endotoxaemia (periphery may be warm)
Heart failure
   myocardial infarction
   pulmonary embolus
   cardiac tamponade
   bacteraemia
Neurogenic—sympathetic inhibition, intracranial haemorrhage
Miscellaneous—electrolyte and fluid loss (vomiting and diarrhoea)
   Treatment is designed, with regard to aetiology:
1. to increase cardiac output by increasing blood volume or by using inotropic agents
2. to raise $P_aO_2$ by increasing $F_1O_2$ and may require IPPV
3. to eliminate infection
4. to sustain renal function
   In the majority of situations the cause can be determined by central venous pressure measurement and measurement of systolic blood pressure.
Relative or absolute hypovolaemia
   Low CVP    low systemic blood pressure
Pump failure
   High CVP    low systemic blood pressure

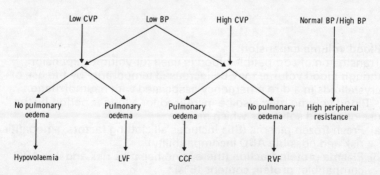

**Fig 5.1** Differentiation of the causes of poor perfusion

## ASSESSMENT AND TREATMENT AND HYPOVOLAEMIA

To assess the magnitude of hypovolaemia a dynamic assessment of central venous pressure (CVP) must be made—a volume of fluid (100–200 ml of saline) is infused quickly and the response of the CVP monitored—no change in CVP suggests a gross state of hypovolaemia (Fig 5.2a).

A rise in CVP which is transient and falls quickly (Fig 5.2b) indicates a less severe state, and a large rise in CVP with a slow fall (Fig 5.2c) indicates an adequately filled cardiovascular system. Several litres of fluid may be required to replace a volume deficit.

After the first testing of the circulatory status with saline, a colloid of longer intravascular persistence is indicated. If the cause of the perfusion failure is hypovolaemia, then heart rate, blood pressure, urine output and temperature will all respond quickly to adequate fluid replacement. The adequacy of fluid replacement may be confirmed by identifying the response to further aliquots of fluid.

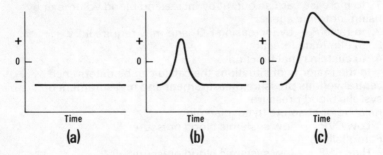

**Fig 5.2** Dynamic testing of the central venous pressure

### Blood volume expansion
Transfusion of compatible blood is used for volume expansion, though blood volume may be increased temporarily by the use of crystalloids in a dire emergency associated with haemorrhage.

Blood volume may also be increased for a longer period by the use of colloid solutions which include;
a) Fresh frozen plasma (this includes all clotting factors, a hepatitis risk and possible ABO incompatibility)
b) Plasma protein fraction (there is no hepatitis risk and it is ABO compatible; protein content 15%)
c) Single donor plasma (this includes all stable clotting factors; Hepatitis is a possible risk and also ABO incompatibility)
d) Albumin (25% albumin in water; oncotic pressure = oncotic pressure of plasma × 5)

e) Dextrans (dextran 70, with a molecular weight of 70 000, exceeds the renal threshold and has a water-binding capacity of 20–25 ml/g. It is therefore an effective plasma expander: however, anaphylactoid reactions are possible).

f) Gelatin (gelatin has a molecular weight of approximately 30 000 and a water-binding capacity of 14 ml.g$^{-1}$. Anaphylactoid reactions are possible).

## ASSESSMENT AND MANAGEMENT OF PUMP FAILURE

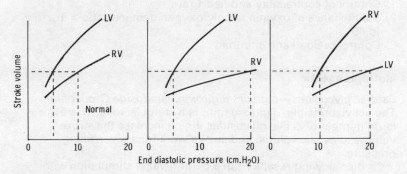

**Fig 5.3** End diastolic pressure/stroke volume relations in the heart

The outflow of blood from the 'right' heart must equal the outflow from the 'left' heart.

Right SV × HR = CO = HR × left SV

Right SV = Left SV

It can be seen from the above diagrams that different end diastolic pressures (roughly equivalent to CVP, and left atrial pressure) are required to produce the same stroke volume in the two ventricles. In the normal heart a CVP of 10 cmH$_2$O will produce an equivalent right ventricular stroke volume to that produced by 5 cmH$_2$O in the left ventricle. A failing right ventricle requires a greater CVP to produce the same stroke volume, in left ventricular failure a higher driving pressure is also required, this unfortunately may have other consequences. If the driving pressure required to produce an adequate stroke volume/cardiac output is greater than 20 cmH$_2$O then the oncotic pressure of the pulmonary circulation is exceeded and pulmonary oedema occurs.

Pump failure can therefore be differentiated by the CVP and BP determination and the absence or presence of pulmonary oedema.

Catheterization of the pulmonary artery using a flow directed catheter, in addition to measurement of the pulmonary artery pressure and cardiac output measurement, by determining the pulmonary capillary wedge pressure (PCWP) allows the filling pressures of the left atrium and therefore the left ventricular end diastolic pressure (LVEDP) to be estimated. In the presence of severe left-sided heart failure the PCWP exceeds 20 mmHg but is less than the LVEDP. Pulmonary artery catheterization also permits the arteriovenous oxygen difference to be determined. A raised or a reduced cardiac output are suggested by a value less than 3 vols % and greater than 6 vols % respectively.

The management of 'pump' failure has several important facets:
1. Control of contractility and heart rate
2. Maintenance of oxygen supply/oxygen demand ratio > 1 (p 45)
3. Control preload and afterload

**Inotropic agents**

*Cardiac glycosides—digoxin, digitoxin, lanatoside C, ouabain*
The active principle, digitoxigenin, is a sterol lactone. There are a large number of active glycosides which increase the stroke volume, diastolic volume and stroke work for a given filling pressure.

Cardiac slowing results from a central vagal stimulation with peripheral potentiation of the vagal effect. In addition there is reduced atrio-ventricular conduction.

Inhibition of membrane ATP occurs, thus inhibiting the sodium pump allowing sodium to flow into the cell and potassium to flow out. The increase in intracellular sodium may facilitate the entry of calcium with the resultant inotropic effect. On the other hand the fall in intracellular potassium slows a–v conduction and sensitises the sinus node to vagal stimulation.

*Dopamine*
Dopamine is produced from DOPA in the penultimate step of the biosynthesis of noradrenaline. The biosynthesis of noradrenaline from tyrosine includes the conversion of dopa to dopamine. Dopamine is released by dopaminergic fibres and stimulates alpha and beta adrenoceptors and dopamine receptors.

Dopamine infused at 2–5 $\mu$g.kg$^{-1}$.min$^{-1}$ produces vasodilatation of the mesenteric and renal vessels. At 5–10 $\mu$g.kg$^{-1}$.min$^{-1}$ it has an inotropic effect and increases the heart rate. A dose of > 15 $\mu$g.kg$^{-1}$.min$^{-1}$ produces vasoconstriction.

*Dobutamine*
A beta-adrenergic inotrope, does not produce a tachycardia.

## Oxygenation

Circulatory failure is generally associated with hypoxaemia. The decreased pulmonary blood flow associated with a reduced blood volume may lead to the dead space increasing up to 80% of the tidal volume. Increased oxygen extraction at the periphery results in further desaturation of mixed venous blood with increased arterial hypoxaemia. Oxygen administration is essential and indeed the increased alveolar ventilation associated with IPPV may outweigh its disadvantages.

## Vasodilators (arterial and venous)

Vasodilating drugs may significantly increase vascular capacity and thereby endanger cerebral and coronary artery blood flow. However vasodilation reduces the afterload, i.e. the pressure opposing the heart (systemic vascular resistance).

If in spite of a normal or raised blood pressure tissue perfusion is poor the use of a vasodilating agent may improve peripheral perfusion by reducing vasoconstriction. Chlorpromazine (1–2 mg repeated at 5-minute intervals) or sodium nitroprusside, which primarily reduces afterload, are useful in the presence of a raised blood pressure and a low PCWP, whereas glyceryl trinitrate primarily a venodilator reduces preload and is useful in patients with myocardial ischaemia (the end diastolic pressure is lower and therefore so is the ventricular wall tension—myocardial perfusion is thus enhanced).

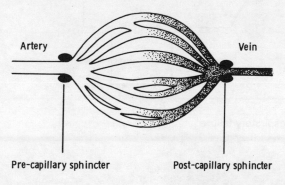

Artery                                             Vein

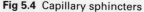

Pre-capillary sphincter          Post-capillary sphincter

**Fig 5.4** Capillary sphincters

The precapillary sphincter constricts in response to catecholamines and the postcapillary sphincter in response to hypoxaemia and an associated fall in pH. Constriction of the precapillary sphincter will ultimately produce contraction of the postcapillary sphincter because of reduced oxygen delivery. Constricted peripheral arterioles, with pre- and postcapillary sphincter constriction, by further reducing tissue perfusion increase further the tissue hypoxia. Relaxation of the arterioles by using vasoactive drugs, accompanied by efficient oxygenation, will cause relaxation of the venous sphincters. If this does not occur there is pooling of blood within the capillary network.

The reduction in peripheral resistance resulting from alpha blockade may well improve left ventricular function in that the afterload is decreased; however a fall in blood pressure—particularly diastolic—also reduces oxygen delivery to the myocardium.

## RESPIRATORY FAILURE

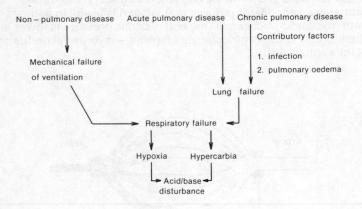

Fig 5.5 Respiratory failure

## Non-pulmonary disease

*CNS depression*
Hypoxaemia
Hypercarbia
Hypotension
Raised ICP
Infection
Drugs
Trauma
Tumour

*Spinal cord disease*
Poliomyelitis
Acute polyneuritis
Demyelination

*Nerve and muscle disorders*

Peripheral neuropathy
Muscular dystrophy

*Disorders of neuromuscular transmission*
Myasthenia gravis
Botulinus toxin
Neuromuscular junction blockers
Aminoglycoside antibiotics
Relaxant drugs

*Chest wall*
Kyphoscoliosis
Fractured ribs

*Pleural space*
Pneumothorax
Haemothorax
Pleural effusion

ACUTE PULMONARY DISEASE
Broncho pneumonia
Lobar pneumonia

CHRONIC PULMONARY DISEASE
Chronic bronchitis
Emphysema
Pulmonary fibrosis
Pneumoconiosis
Bronchial asthma

Hypoxia may occur with or without hypercarbia and may be related to either respiratory or cardiac disease. For a classification of respiratory disorders see pages 28–36.
Upper or lower airway disease (tracheal obstruction/asthma)
Excess secretions (consolidation)
$\dot{V}_A/\dot{Q}_C$ disturbance (atelectasis/pulmonary emboli/shock)

## Oxygen therapy
Hypoxia is the indication for oxygen administration and is usually without hazard. However, the patient whose ventilatory drive depends largely on a low oxygen tension and the patient who requires prolonged administration of a very high concentration of oxygen are at risk.

The classic 'blue bloater' is not common but oxygen therapy may reduce the hypoxic respiratory drive and thus lead, if undiagnosed, to $CO_2$ narcosis. The inspired oxygen concentration must be titrated, generally between 25 and 30% which substantially increases $O_2$ saturation but with only a minimal increase in $P_aO_2$ and hence $P_aCO_2$.

Oxygen toxicity may not always result from breathing high partial pressures of oxygen, however the administration of high oxygen concentrations to premature babies may rapidly lead to retrolental fibroplasia. Collapse of alveoli as oxygen is absorbed is a more common problem associated with a high $F_IO_2$ than damage to the alveolar cells.

Many factors may protect the patient from the fatal oxygen toxicity syndrome. Drugs and intermittent exposure to lower oxygen concentrations are notable examples. However the patient treated with IPPV may be particularly at risk. It is less easy to achieve a high $F_IO_2$ when the patient breathes through a mask. Correction of other factors may reduce the need for an excessive inspired oxygen concentration. Hypoproteinaemia affects membrane integrity and pyrexia influences oxygen transfer and requirements. Active cooling may be used to reduce oxygen consumption and may protect the vital organs, the brain in particular.

## Bronchodilators

1. Sympathomimetic drugs (beta agonist activity)
   adrenaline, salbutamol, isoprenaline, terbutaline, orciprenaline, ephedrine
2. Phosphodiesterase inhibitors (increase intracellular c-AMP)
   aminophylline, choline, theophylinate
3. Steroid agents (anti inflammatory effect, reduces capillary permeability and increases intracellular c-AMP)
   hydrocortisone, prednisolone
4. Anti allergy drugs (stabilises mast cell membrane, preventing the release of bronchospasmic agents)
   disodium cromoglycate
   ketotifen

## Respiratory stimulants

Respiratory stimulants are indicated when the respiratory drive is insufficient to prevent a progressively increasing $P_aCO_2$ (hypoxia can be treated with oxygen).

These should not be used in the patient who is obviously distressed and working maximally in an attempt to maintain gaseous exchange, e.g. the patient in status asthmaticus.

Doxapram is a frequently used respiratory stimulant and has a place in the management of those patients with respiratory depression due to centrally acting drugs such as the barbiturates or narcotics.

## Intermittent positive pressure ventilation
When spontaneous respiratory activity is insufficient mechanical inflation of the lungs is indicated.
1. Maintenance of the airway
   Non-irritant endotracheal tubes, nasal or oral, are used.
   *Nasal* — less relative movement, easy to keep mouth clean, patient can drink and eat; however, greater length, narrower bore and therefore greater resistance and tendency to collapse and cause obstruction. Difficulty due to narrow bore with aspiration of secretions. Damage to nasal mucosa is possible.
   *Oral* — moves with swallowing or chewing—not easy to fix securely, mouth toilet is more difficult, lower resistance and aspiration of secretions is fairly easy
   *Tracheostomy*—with modern non-irritant endotracheal tubes with low pressure cuffs it might be argued that tracheostomy is no longer indicated because of its attendant dangers—infection and haemorrhage. However, the patient may tolerate a tracheostomy tube when an oral or nasal tube is not tolerated.
2. Selection of respiratory pattern
   a) low tidal volume, high rate
   b) high tidal volume, low rate
   c) high tidal volume, high rate
   d) PEEP/inspiratory hold
   There are many permutations. The aim is to produce the greatest rise in $P_aO_2$ or $S_aO_2$ for the least rise in mean intrathoracic pressure.
3. Humidification—page 185.
4. Monitoring of respiratory parameters by the nursing and medical staff is mandatory and alarm systems are necessary to detect mechanical faults.

*Non-specific therapy*
Antibiotics
Physiotherapy
Mucolytic agents
Cooling
   The aim of cooling is to reduce oxygen requirements so that the amount delivered to the tissues is sufficient to meet their needs.
   Core and surface temperatures must be measured.
   The patient must be efficiently sedated and paralysed.
   Peripheral vasodilation and reduction in shivering (chlorpromazine and muscle relaxation) allows easier heat exchange.

Heating devices are turned off, e.g. blood warmers and heated humidifiers, and ice packs are placed over the carotid arteries, the groins and in the axillae. Cold sponging and fans are used to increase heat lost by evaporation. A heat-exchange blanket can be used to maintain the state of hypothermia without the patient being continually wet.

Large core/surface temperature differences are hazardous—movement of limbs may cause a large amount of cold blood to reach the heart and cause ventricular fibrillation (VF).

Active cooling is stopped at 32°C or above, as further cooling may occur (the 'after drop') and may cause the temperature to fall a further 2–3°. Ventricular fibrillation is likely below 28°C

Rewarming should be allowed to occur naturally: the slightest excess heat may damage the skin.

## Discontinuance of ventilation

Most patients can be weaned easily and quickly from the ventilator but some require weaning to be a prolonged and gradual process and indeed present a protracted problem. The patient's condition must be optimal, no heart failure, no pyrexia, no anaemia and no abdominal splinting.

Bronchospasm and secretions must be minimal. A vital capacity of at least 10 ml.kg$^{-1}$ is thought necessary to achieve weaning also a VD/VT ratio of less than 0.6 and an ability to generate at least – 20 cmH$_2$O pressure on inspiration.

*Techniques*
a) Intermittant spontaneous respiration—possible danger of severe hypoxia
b) Triggering—patient and machine often poorly synchronised
c) Intermittant mandatory ventilation (IMV)—there is no real evidence of shortened weaning time; however it is safe
d) Mandatory minute ventilation—not in common usage—it has a theoretical advantage over IMV, in that the minute ventilation is controlled
e) Continuous positive airway pressure (CPAP)—this may be used alone, or in conjunction with IMV and may assist weaning

## Blood gases—their interpretation

A $P_a$o$_2$ of less than 5 kPa is considered to be hypoxaemic.
    Apart from pathological processes, age and altitude alter $P_a$o$_2$.
A $P_a$co$_2$ of greater than 8 kPa is considered to be hypercarbic
A $P_a$co$_2$ between 6.5 and 8 kPa may be normal for the patient with chronic respiratory disease.
1. Oxygen therapy is indicated if the $P_a$o$_2$ is less than 5 kPa and an increase in alveolar ventilation is generally necessary if the $P_a$co$_2$ is greater than 8 kPa.

2. Various degrees of oxygen therapy are needed between a $P_aO_2$ of 5 kPa and 7 kPa, and an increase in alveolar ventilation may be necessary if the $P_aCO_2$ lies between 6.5 kPa and 8 kPa in the patient with acute respiratory failure.
3. Oxygen therapy with a $P_aO_2$ greater than 7 kPa is not essential unless there is concommitant ischaemic vascular disease. The practice of maintaining normal or above normal $P_aO_2$ levels by using high concentrations of inspired oxygen may not be beneficial.

## RENAL FAILURE

Renal failure exists if the serum creatinine is raised. Urea may be raised for other reasons; dehydration, catabolism or blood in the intestine in addition to renal failure.

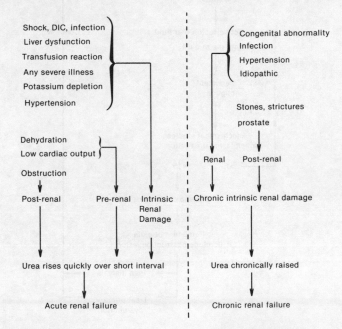

**Fig 5.6** Renal failure

The diagnosis of acute renal failure depends almost entirely on the rapid changes in the biochemistry of the patient as the urine flow may be normal, high or low. In the patient with acute renal failure signs and symptoms of uraemia are a late sign.

Patients with chronic renal failure may suddenly deteriorate and are usually admitted to hospital in uraemia.

URAEMIA: Lethargy, fits, coma, thirst, vomiting, anorexia, haematemesis, air hunger, hiccough

A systematic approach should be made to the differential diagnosis of acute renal failure but the uraemic patient should firstly be treated, and then the differential diagnosis considered.

## Investigation of acute renal failure

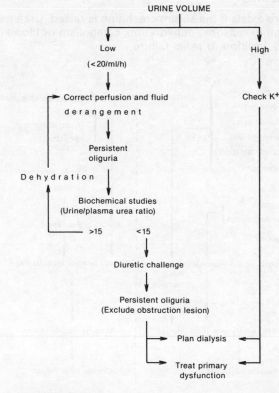

**Fig 5.7** Acute renal failure

## Management
1. Treat primary disorder if possible
2. Preserve veins
3. Avoid infection
4. Careful fluid balance (weigh bed)
5. Maintain nutritional status (starvation accentuates uraemia)
6. Dialysis
7. Correction of anaemia
8. Maintain protein levels

## Dialysis

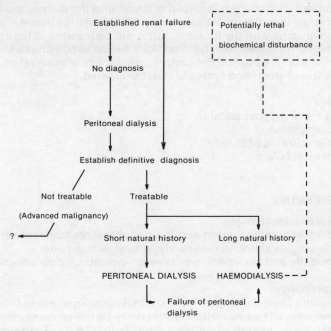

**Fig 5.8** Dialysis

## Peritoneal dialysis
Diffusion and osmosis across the peritoneum—a semi-permeable membrane.

Small molecules move freely according to concentration gradients.

Water molecules move in accordance with the laws of osmosis.

Dialysis fluids are designed for specific purposes—their osmolality determines the amount of water removed, and their electrolyte concentrations the amount of electrolytes removed.

Hazards
Infection
Hypovolaemia—removal of too much water
Hyperglycaemia—dialysate osmolarity determined mainly by its
                    dextrose concentration.
Haemorrhage
Diaphragmatic splinting
Hypoproteinaemia

*Haemodialysis*
Diffusion, osmosis and ultrafiltration. Ultrafiltration is the result of
pressurising blood in contact with the artificial semipermeable
membrane so that water is forced through into the dialysis fluid.
   For short-term haemodialysis a shunt is inserted between artery
and vein, usually on the forearm, but it can be inserted at the ankle.
   For long-term haemodialysis an A–V fistula is constructed.
Dialysis is tailored to suit the patient;, electrolyte concentration,
extraction of water and timing are all considered.

Hazards
Hypotension/hypovolaemia
Anticoagulation
Infection/clotting of shunt
Mechanical failure

## LIVER FAILURE

### Cardiovascular changes
The cardiac output is raised and the peripheral resistance lowered.
Arterio-venous shunting occurs. Hypotension occurs not
infrequently and persistant hypotension indicates a poor prognosis.

### Mental changes
Fluctuating mental changes, from normal consciousness to coma.
Octopamine, a false neurotransmitter, may be the cause of coma,
and excess circulating ammonia a contributing factor. Tryptophan,
which is found to be increased, is converted to serotonin which can
also induce sleep. (The increase in free fatty acids that occurs
affects brain uptake of typtophan and thus may also influence the
mental changes).
   There are many other non specific factors–hypotension, hypoxia
and hypoglycaemia, the latter possibly resulting from the increase
in insulin levels that occur in chronic liver disease. These mental
changes associated with coma are reversible but metabolic brain
damage can occur resulting in convulsions and cerebral oedema,
which may not be reversible.

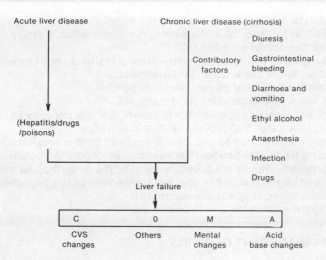

**Fig 5.9** Liver failure

## Acid/base changes
Ammonia stimulates ventilation to produce respiratory alkalosis.
Renal problems, antacids or gastric drainage may produce a
metabolic alkalosis.

## Other effects
Renal failure, the hepatorenal syndrome, may occur (an acute
tubular necrosis or shunting of blood from the cortex to the
medulla). Uraemia may be the result of the absorption of excessive
nitrogenous compounds from the gut—commonly blood.
   A coagulopathy occurs, clotting factors are decreased and the
prothrombin time is increased.
   Pulmonary dysfunction, infection, oedema and 'shock lung' leads
to hypoxia.

## Management
Monitoring of ECG, BP, and CVP is essential.
Dextrose is the safest intravenous fluid.
Avoid absorption of toxic material from the bowel by the use of
magnesium sulphate enemas or lactulose.
No sedation should be prescribed even if the patient is restless.
Endotracheal intubation may be necessary to prevent aspiration.
   (Duration of action of suxamethonium may be marginally
   prolonged)
   (Avoid gallamine—renal failure will prolong its action)
IPPV is necessary if the patient is hypoxic due to hypoventilation or
convulsions.

Electrolyte derangement—commonly hypokalaemia; may require large K$^+$ supplements, and a severe metabolic alkalosis may require correction with N/6 HCl.
Hypovolaemia is badly tolerated—treat adequately with careful attention to the cardiovascular parameters.
Intropic support may be required—dopamine.
Treat renal failure as described on p 162.
Peritoneal dialysis is preferable to haemodialysis because of the poor tolerance of hypovolaemia. Avoid diuretics.
Cimetidine is needed to reduce incidence of gastric erosions.
Bleeding from oesophageal varices may be controlled by using a Sengstaken–Blakemore tube (injection of the oesophageal varices seems to be the current vogue, but transection of the oesophagus is the definitive surgical management).
Anticipate, search for and treat infection.

## THE MANAGEMENT OF BURNS

1. Fluid balance
2. Respiratory care
3. General management

### 1. Fluid balance
Assess % area of burns (Wallace rule of 9s)

| | |
|---|---|
| Head | 1 × 9% |
| Arms | 2 × 9% |
| Legs | 4 × 9% |
| Trunk | 4 × 9% |
| | 11 × 9% × 99% |
| Genitalia | 1% |
| | 100% |

Plasma is given, according to a formula based on the % burn, and body-weight (Mount Vernon formula), in a given period of time.

$$\frac{\% \text{ burn} \times \text{wt (kg)}}{2} = \text{ml/period}$$

the time periods are 4, 4, 4, 6, 6 and 12 hours.
The PCV can be used to determine the blood volume deficit

$$\frac{\text{Deficit}}{\text{(litres)}} = \frac{\text{Blood volume}}{\text{(ht/wt nomogram)}} - \frac{\text{Blood vol.} \times \text{normal PCV}}{\text{observed PCV}}$$

and the blood volume deficit is then replaced by more plasma.
If the PCV is normal a plasma/saline mixture (50:50) is given.

Evaporation of fluid from burns may be extremely high, up to 8 litres per day, and this must be replaced.

## 2.  Respiratory care

A respiratory burn must be suspected if the face, oral mucosa or nasal hairs are burnt. The larynx, trachea and main bronchi are damaged by heat but the bronchioles are affected mainly by carbon particles or chemical irritants. Bronchospasm and pulmonary oedema are the major results of respiratory burns. The bronchospasm is unresponsive to bronchodilators; steroids and humidification may help. Pulmonary oedema is controlled by diuretics, digitalisation and intermittent positive pressure respiration. Pneumonic changes inevitably occur and the mortality rate is high.

Tracheotomy may be necessary but some think that it precipitates pulmonary oedema.

Blood gas analysis should be carried out as frequently as the clinical condition of the patient dictates and the carbon monoxide level should also be monitored.

## 3.  General management

a) The haemoglobin, packed cell volume and urea and electrolytes are measured as frequently as necessary to determine fluid requirements.

[Na$^+$] may be used as indicator of the state of hydration.

b) X-ray the chest daily

c) Urinary catherisation if > 30% burn, a good urine output must be maintained to 'wash out' free Hb from the circulation and kidneys

d) Artificial alimentation

e) Bacterial monitoring of burnt areas

f) Tetanus toxoid

g) Environmental temperature and humidity should be high, 90°F (32°C), 40% humidity

Heat is lost by evaporation of fluid from large raw areas. This heat loss can be reduced by enclosing burnt limbs in polythene bags and by maintaining a high humidity. The calories lost by evaporation must be replaced by hyperalimentation.

h) Surgical management—escharotomies, grafting and dressing with Famazine

i) Analgesia is required for the frequent dressing of burns and may be produced by a 50:50 nitrous oxide/oxygen mixture, methoxyflurane, trichloroethylene or by enflurane. Patient acceptance of enflurane has been found to be high. Verbal contact is maintained and the patient can stand. Enflurane is not unpleasant to inhale. Ketamine is popular and so are intravenous opiates but in children, and in patients with few veins, inhalational methods are preferable.

j)  Anaesthesia is required for major procedures—the only drug
    that may cause problems is suxamethonium: a rise in
    potassium concentration could possibly cause a cardiac arrest.
    Many centres routinely use suxamethonium to facilitate
    intubation and if the potassium level is normal there is probably
    little danger.
      Repeated anaesthetics may be required and the choice of
    agents should reflect this possibility.

## NUTRITIONAL SUPPORT OF THE ILL PATIENT

Following major trauma or surgery, muscle tissue undergoes
catabolism which increases urinary nitrogen. This loss is not
affected by nutrition but feeding high-energy, high-protein diets
leads to a deposition of protein, partially compensating for the
endogenous loss. A negative nitrogen balance occurs because the
anabolic processes producing protein in the liver require amino
acids provided by a greater amount of peripheral protein, a greater
turnover of albumin occurs, fibrinogen levels rise, IgM levels rise
and the concentrations of other proteins rise, all the result of
increased protein synthesis.

  The nitrogenous losses are maximal between the fifth and
seventh days, but the degree of catabolism is less with increasing
age, less in females and less if the patient has previously been in a
state of undernutrition.

  Feeding a patient following 'trauma' may reduce the expected
weight loss by 70%. If the patient is not fed, death may be due to
starvation rather than the initial surgical or traumatic insult.

  Morbidity may be reduced by adequate nutrition. If the gut is
intact and functioning the route of choice is enteral, the alternate
route is intravenous.

### Enteral nutrition

Liquid feed taken enterally avoids many complications associated
with the intravenous route. Patients with oesophageal strictures
may be fed enterally, those incapable of swallowing or having no
desire to eat or drink may be fed via a fine-bore nasogastric tube.
Fine bore tubes are well tolerated and cause minimal trauma to
mucosa and enable adequate volumes to be given either by gravity
feed or by roller pump. The feed may contain whole protein,
peptides or free amino acids, those patients with a reduced
proteolytic or absorptive capacity should be given the latter, termed
'elemental' diets.

  Diarrhoea is unlikely if the concentration of the feed is gradually
built up over several days. If it occurs, it may be controlled by
codeine phosphate but lactose intolerance should not be
overlooked and a lactose-free feed should be instituted.

## Parenteral nutrition
Subclavian/internal jugular catheters tunnelled below the skin (see p 113) are the percutaneous venous routes of choice. Lipid solutions are now rarely used. The nitrogen requirements are given in the form of amino acids and the calories in the form of dextrose. The amino acid solutions available may be classified in terms of their ability to deliver nitrogen. (They are complex solutions and the reasons for their composition is beyond the scope of this book.) Once the desired amount of nitrogen, in g/24h has been determined the appropriate solution is selected. Dextrose is given either separately or in a combined solution—large-volume bags (usually 3 l) are now available for each 24 h—which reduces contamination by reducing the number of insertions of administration sets into the highly nutritious medium for bacterial growth.

There are two ways to determine the amount of nitrogen and dextrose that are required.

1. A calculation of nitrogen losses—this method, although giving a precise value, involves a delay in that the results are always at least 24 h out of date, usually more.

2. An assessment of calorie requirements, and then the calculation of the appropriate nitrogen needs. Calorie requirements can be determined from nitrogen needs and vice-versa, however, the 'kcal/g nitrogen' ratio varies with the patient's clinical condition: in the non-catabolic patient the ratio may be 250:1, and in the catabolic 150:1.

An insulin infusion may be required to control blood sugar levels, and to reduce urinary losses of sugar, and the infusion rate may need to be high, as insulin resistance occurs. The blood sugar requires measuring hourly and adjustments must be made to the insulin infusion rate—sliding scales exist but the scale of choice should be designed to prevent large swings in blood glucose levels (see p 170).

Water and electrolyte balance must be maintained—rarer minerals may need to be given.

## Monitoring the patient
Weight
Nitrogen balance—blood and urinary urea
Electrolyte estimation
Plasma proteins
Liver function tests
Blood cultures if pyrexial
Acid/base status
Blood sugar

## BLOOD GLUCOSE CONTROL

*A M J Woolfson, City Hospital, Nottingham*
Assuming insulin administered with a syringe pump
*Blood glucose,*

| Blood glucose, mmol.l$^{-1}$ | | Action |
|---|---|---|
| < 4.0 | | Turn down by 1.0 ml/h |
| 4.0 – 6.9 | | Turn down by 0.5 ml/h |
| 7.0 – 10.9 | | Infusion rate unchanged |
| 11.0 – 15.0 | If lower than previous test | Infusion rate unchanged |
| | If higher than previous test | Turn up by 0.5 ml/h |
| > 15.0 | If lower than previous test | Same rate |
| | If higher than previous test | Turn up by 1.0 ml/h |

If rate reaches O, or 0.5 ml/h, halve concentration in syringe and restart at 0.5 ml/h

If the rate reaches 4.5 or 5 ml/h, double concentration in syringe and restart at 2.5 ml/h.

## MANAGEMENT OF POISONING

### Assessment
Name of drug(s), amount taken, time taken
Neurological status
    Level of consciousness (ability to protect the airway)
    Confusion/restlessness/fits
    Psychiatric assessment
    Thermoregulation
Cardiovascular status
    Blood pressure
    Peripheral perfusion
    Myocardial irritability
Respiratory status
    Alveolar ventilation
    Safety of airway
Hepatic function—is drug hepatotoxic?
Renal function—is drug nephrotoxic?
Neuro-muscular function—is drug anticholinergic?
Fore-gut integrity—is drug caustic?

### Supportive measures
1. Protect airway if necessary—if an endotracheal tube can be passed without sedation or relaxation then one should be passed as the airway is obviously in danger

2. Intravenous infusion—fluids are given as necessary to maintain blood volume/perfusion—a central venous line may be necessary
3. Intermittent positive pressure ventilation if hypoxia or hypercapnia exists
4. Control of cardiac dysrhythmias
5. Temperature regulating blankets as necessary
6. Control of convulsions

**Specific measures**
The aim is to reduce drug effect, absorption and enhance excretion.
1. Antidotes
   Opiates—naloxone
   Iron preparations—desferrioxamine
   Cyanide—Kelacyanor (dicobalt edetate)
2. Gastric lavage—the aim is to remove any remaining drug from the stomach. The time elapsed between ingestion and lavage is important and may make lavage irrelevant. Assessment of airway security is important before attempting lavage.
3. Emetics, particularly salt-water, may be hazardous. Oesophageal rupture and fluid imbalance, with salt water, may result.
4. Enhancement of excretion
   *Forced diuresis*
   Maintenance of urinary output will allow a continuous elimination of the drug. This is achieved by infusion of saline and dextrose together with a diuretic. CVP control is advisable, with meticulous attention to fluid balance. Altering the pH of urine changes the ionization of the drug present in the tubules and if the ionization is increased reabsorption is reduced.
   *Salicylates, barbiturates*—alkaline urine
   *Amphetamines, quinine, fenfluramine*—acidic urine
   *Peritoneal dialysis*—see page 163
   *Haemodialysis*—see page 164

**Barbiturates**
Severe overdose—coma
              —ventilatory depression
              —hypotension
Treatment      —intubation
              —IPPV
              —plasma expansion
              —forced diuresis
Short acting—3 $mg.dl^{-1}$ >4 $mg.dl^{-1}$ haemodialyse
Long acting—10 $mg.dl^{-1}$ >15 $mg.dl^{-1}$ haemodialyse

**Salicylates**
Child—3 mg.dl$^{-1}$
Adult—50 mg.dl$^{-1}$
Severe overdose—conscious
  —severe acidosis
  —reduced prothrombin level
  —hypokalaemia
  —hyponatraemia (hypernatraemia may result from attempts to raise pH with sodium bicarbonate in the presence of a very severe acidosis)
Treatment    —gastric lavage or induced vomiting
  —forced alkaline diuresis (mannitol or frusemide)
  —increase potassium input with infusion fluids
  —intravenous vitamin K
  —hyperventilation may require to be controlled using IPPV
  —peritoneal dialysis if plasma concentration > 100 mg.dl$^{-1}$

**Paracetamol**
Overdose —conscious
  —hepatic damage—> 300 $\mu$g. ml$^{-1}$ at 4 h
         > 75 $\mu$g. ml$^{-1}$ at 12 h
  —prothrombin time prolonged
  —hypoglycaemia
  —metabolic acidosis
  —acute renal failure
Treatment—cysteamine may prevent hepatic damage if given within 10 hours as may:
      iv. N-acetylcysteine
      gastric lavage
      reduced further absorption with charcoal and cholestyramine
      charcoal column haemoperfusion

**Dextropropoxyphene**
—Respiratory depression, coma and cardiovascular collapse
—Naloxone antagonizes the effect of dextroproxyphene but its own effect is of shorter duration than the agonist and may therefore require to be given in repeated doses

**Phenothiazines**
Overdose —drowsiness
  —coma
  —respiratory depression
  —hypotension

Treatment—gastric lavage
 —vasopressors or plasma expander may be required to combat hypotension
 —IPPV may be required

**Tricyclics**
Overdose —coma
 —respiratory depression
 —convulsions
 —cardiac dysrhythmias which include tachycardia, atrial flutter, atrio- and intra-ventricular block
Treatment—Phentolamine if hypertension occurs
 —Symptomatic treatment of convulsions and cardiac dysrhythmia

**Paraquat**
Overdose —progressive and lethal pulmonary fibrosis.
Treatment—prevent further absorption—500 ml of 30% Fuller's earth and 5% magnesium
 —haemoperfusion over activated charcoal or carbon exchange resin
 —d-propranolol competes with paraquat binding sites
 —forced diuresis or haemodialysis
 —lower $P_aO_2$ to 5.5–8 kPa. The toxic effect of paraquat is similar to that of oxygen toxicity and thus high inspired oxygen concentrations should be avoided.

**Carbon monoxide**
Treatment
Raise $F_IO_2$ to 100% or treat with hyperbaric oxygen
Search for other drugs and treat accordingly
Use mannitol if there are signs of raised intracranial pressure

**Methyl alcohol**
Alkalis are use to combat intense acidosis due to formation of formic acid.
Ethanol may delay the oxidation of methanol and hence reduce the acidosis.

**Carbon tetrachloride**
Hepatotoxicity—management depends on severity
Nephrotoxicity—haemodialysis necessary
Cardiac dysrhythmias
Pulmonary oedema

**Organophosphorous insecticides—anticholinesterases**
Overdose —pulmonary oedema
—convulsions
Treatment—Atropine may be given as an infusion; however it may
have to be given repeatedly, intravenously in 2 mg
boluses at 10-minute intervals, until the secretions are
controlled
—Pralidoxime chloride 1–2 g i.v. (500 mg.min$^{-1}$)
—Anticonvulsants—diazepam 0.3 mg.kg$^{-1}$ (5 mg.min$^{-1}$)

## DIAGNOSIS OF BRAIN DEATH

1. The cause of the coma should be known
2. Hypothermia and drug effects should be excluded
3. Brain function should be assessed at least twice at 12-hourly
   intervals
   a) No spontaneous activity
   b) No abnormal posturing
   c) No epileptic jerking
   d) No brain stem reflexes
      (i) No pupillary response to light
      (ii) No corneal reflex
      (iii) No gag reflex
      (iv) No oculo-cephalic reflexes
      (v) No oculo-vestibular reflexes
   e) No spontaneous respiration

$P_{a}co_2$ and $P_{a}o_2$ must be normal. Oxygenation with 100% $O_2$ is
then carried out for at least 7 minutes.

An oxygen insufflation catheter is passed into the trachea and
apnoeic diffusion oxygenation allowed. Respiratory activity is then
noted.

The legal implications of terminating treatment vary from country
to country. Brain stem death—as described above—implies that
the patient is dead and further treatment is irrelevant.

# 6. Equipment

## THE ANAESTHETIC MACHINE

Many configurations of anaesthetic machine are in use. Basically, fresh gases are delivered at 60 lb.in$^{-2}$ (4 bar) from cylinders or pipelines and the flow is controlled by metering the gases through flow meters (rotameters). The gases may then be passed through a vaporiser and thence either via a reservoir bag, usually of 2 l capacity, (spontaneous ventilation) and various systems to a patient or to a ventilator (controlled ventilation).

The pressure rise in the system resulting from obstruction to the outlet of the anaesthetic machine may cause damage to the rotameters and vaporisers. These may however be protected by a pressure relief valve opening at 35 kPa (350 cmH$_2$O). Commonly-used ventilators driven by the anaesthetic gases only require 20 kPa to function.

## BULK GAS STORAGE

### Liquid oxygen
Liquid oxygen is transported by road in double-walled spherical containers; the outer wall is constructed from steel and the inner from copper. This type of container, which resembles the Dewar flask and contains enough liquid oxygen to produce 100 000 ft$^3$ on evaporation, is used to 'top-up' the smaller but similarly-designed hospital storage tanks. The liquid oxygen is usually stored at a pressure below 180 lb.in$^{-2}$ and at a temperature maintained lower than the critical figure of $-119°C$.

### Pipelines
Oxygen, nitrous oxide, Entonox, vacuum and compressed air can be provided by pipeline. Connection to the anaesthetic and other apparatus is made by means of flexible hoses and non-interchangeable connectors. The gases may be stored centrally in banks of large cylinders. Auditory and visual alarm devices may be used to give warning of a failure in the pipe supply.

## CYLINDERS

Most cylinders used for storage of gases used in anaesthetic practice are manufactured from molybdenum steel. They have to be strong to withstand rough handling during use and transport.

Three types of mechanical testing are employed: one in every batch or one in every hundred cylinders produced is tested.
1. Tensile test. Tests are made on strips cut longitudinally from finished cylinders. The strips are tensioned until they elongate (yield).
2. Flattening, impact and bend tests. The middle half of an empty cylinder is placed between two compression blocks. The impact and bend tests stress the metal to the point of cracking.
3. Hydraulic and/or pressure test. The cylinder is enclosed in a vessel filled with water and simultaneously the pressure of water within the cylinder is increased. The change in volume of the cylinder on applying and after removal of the internal hydraulic pressure is measured by changes in the level of water in the vessel.

### Identification and marking of cylinders
1. Cylinders are painted externally as follows:

|  | Valve end | Body |
|---|---|---|
| Oxygen | White | Black |
| Nitrous oxide | Blue | Blue |
| Cyclopropane | Orange | Orange |
| Carbon dioxide | Grey | Grey |
| Helium | Brown | Brown |
| Nitrogen | Black | Grey |
| $O_2$ and $CO_2$ | White and grey | Black |
| $O_2$ and He | White and Brown | Grey |
| Air | White and Black | Grey |
| $N_2O/O_2$ | White and Blue | Blue |

2. Each gas cylinder bears a label showing the name of the gas contained in the cylinder
3. The name or chemical symbol is stencilled in paint on the shoulder of the cylinder
4. Cylinder outlet valves have punched on them:
   a) Name of the contained gas
   b) The tare weight
   c) The name of the manufacturer
   d) The cylinder size
   e) A series of dates indicating when the cylinder was subjected to hydraulic testing. Thus 81 ① means the first quarter of 1981. More recently a plastic 'marker', rings retained between the cylinder and the outlet, has been employed for this purpose.
   f) The serial number of the valve and cylinder

5. The cylinder necks have punched on them:
   a) The date of testing
   b) The serial number of the cylinder

**Non-interchangeability**
Non-interchangeable flush-type pin index valves prevent the
connection of cylinders to the wrong yokes or flow meters. These
are fitted to all cylinders up to and including 12 lb water capacity.

Hole Numbers for<br>Index Pins

| | | |
|---|---|---|
| Oxygen | 2 and 5 | |
| Oxygen and $CO_2$ | 2 and 6 | 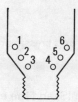 |
| Nitrous Oxide | 3 and 5 | |
| Cyclopropane | 3 and 6 | |

**Fig 6.1** Pin index codes

'Bull-nose' valves are fitted to oxygen cylinders exceeding 48 ft$^3$
capacity. The design of valves is so arranged that they are
non-interchangeable.

| Storage pressures | kg.cm$^{-2}$ |
|---|---|
| Oxygen | 139.2 |
| Nitrous oxide | 44.9 |
| Carbon dioxide | 50.8 |
| Cyclopropane | 4.5 |

## PRESSURE REGULATORS/FLOW RESTRICTORS

**Regulators**
There are several types of regulator available. In a low-pressure
regulator the diaphragm is usually made of rubber or neoprene
whereas in high-pressure regulators the diaphragms are usually
metal. A two stage regulator is used when high flow rates and large
pressure reductions are required.
1. The McKesson regulator.
     High-pressure reduction—metal diaphragm.
     Adjustment can be made by other than a service engineer.
2. The Adam's regulator.
     The input may vary from 2000 lb.in$^{-2}$ (cylinder) to 60 lb.in$^{-2}$
     (pipeline).
     Because of the toggle arrangement, the pressure acting
     against the diaphragm moves the needle in the opposite
     direction thereby occluding the high pressure aperture. The

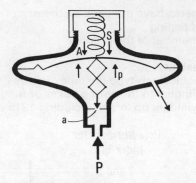

Fig 6.2 Adam's pressure reducing valve

spring (S) and the elastic recoil of the diaphragm, distorted by the low pressure gas, oppose the force exerted by the high pressure gas on the needle.

Thus    $Pa + S = pA$

By altering S pressure reduction can be varied.
Safety pressure release valves are often fitted on the downstream side of a regulator to offer some protection to the patient in case of regulator failure.

### Flow restrictors
Regulators are occasionally omitted when anaesthetic machines are supplied from pipelines at a pressure of 60 lb.in$^{-2}$. Sudden pressure surges at the patient end of the machine are prevented by flow restrictors fitted between the supply and the rotameters.

### CHECKING BULK GAS SUPPLY AND CYLINDERS
1. Check bulk gas warning lights
2. 'One Gas' test—this eliminates the possibility of crossed pressure hoses
   a) Check that the high-pressure gas hose for oxygen is connected to the correct wall outlet or large cylinder regulator and to the oxygen inlet on the anaesthetic machine
   b) Turn on the oxygen source and turn off all other gas sources
   c) After all the other gases have been 'bled' from the machine open all flow-meter controls and check that oxygen only flows
3. Repeat 'one-gas' test for nitrous oxide
4. Test oxygen supply warning device if fitted

5. Check the levels of contents of all cylinders fitted to machines. This also detects leaks and ensures that there is a key to fit each cylinder.
6. Turn off reserve cylinders
7. Turn all wall outlets to ensure that male hose connector is firmly secured in female wall outlets

## MEASUREMENT OF FLOW RATE OF GASES

The devices commonly employed today to meter the flow rate of gases are:
1. The Rotameter—the calibrated glass tube is tapered and contains a cone-shaped float which has oblique notches cut in the rim to encourage its rotation. Inaccuracies may occur if the tube is not vertical, is dirty, or is subjected to static electricity.
2. Ball float meters—these also have a tapered tube which may be monitored vertically or sloping. The Quantiflex gas mixer not only incorporates such a metering device but also enables the oxygen concentration to be preset.
3. The Heidbrink meter—once again the tube is tapered. Here the position of a metal rod is determined by the flow rate.
4. The Forreger meter—this water depression constant orifice meter is still widely used in the USA.

## VAPORISERS

### Non-temperature compensated
1. The 'Boyle' Bottle
2. The Goldman Vaporiser
3. Copper Kettle
4. The Draeger 'Vapor'
5. Bryce-Smith Induction Unit

### Temperature compensated

1. *Continuous flow*
   a) The Fluotec, Ethertec, Tritec, Pentec, Enfluorotec Mark 3
   b) The Halothane 4
   c) The Abingdon Vaporizers
   d) The Penlon
   e) Blease Universal Vaporiser

2. *Draw-over vaporisers*
   a) Ether-pac
   b) Fluo-pac
   c) AE Fluothane Vaporiser
   d) Oxford Miniature Vaporiser (OMV)
   e) Epstein/Macintosh/Oxford (EMO)

*VIC = Vaporiser inside circle*
The patient breathes spontaneously through a vaporiser in the
circle circuit and therefore the resistance to gas flow should be low.
Furthermore as the respired gases are going to pass through the
vaporiser several times the inspired concentration will be higher
than that set on the dial and therefore its efficiency in terms of the
concentration that it can deliver should also be low. Spontaneous
breathing is safer than controlled ventilation. During spontaneous
breathing respiratory depression associated with high dose of
anaesthetic occurs, the minute ventilation is reduced. This reduces
the passage of gas through the vaporiser and hence reduces the
inspired concentration.

*VOC = Vaporiser outside circle*
With the vaporiser outside the circle there is no need for a low
resistance to gas flow. The inspired concentration of vapour is
lower than that set on the dial because the expired gases, of lower
vapour concentration, dilute the vapour in the fresh gas.
Intermittent positive pressure ventilation is not contraindicated.

## BREATHING SYSTEMS

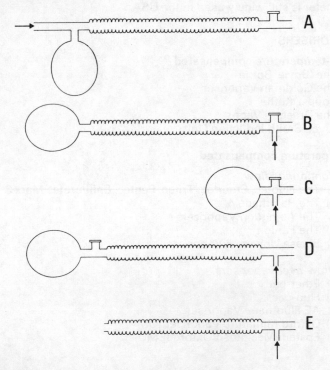

**Fig 6.3** Mapleson's classification of breathing systems

### Without carbon dioxide absorption
Mapleson in 1954 classified the existing breathing systems into five groups, A–E, depending on their characteristic re-breathing properties.

The flow of fresh gas required to prevent re-breathing of $CO_2$ in each type has been determined.

**Table 3**

| Mapleson type | Fresh gas flow to prevent re-breathing of $CO_2$ | | |
|---|---|---|---|
| | Spontaneous ventilation | | Controlled ventilation |
| A. Magill, Lack*[1] | 0.75V | (VA) | Depends on mode of operation[†] |
| B. | 2.0 V | | > 8 1.min$^{-1}$ |
| C. Water's system | 2.0–3.0 V̇ | | > 8 1.min$^{-1}$ |
| D. Bain*[2] | 1.5–2.0 V | | 70 ml.min$^{-1}$kg$^{-1}$ |
| E. Ayres T-piece/Bain*[3] | 1.5–2.0 V | | $(I+(E/I)) \times \dot{V}$ (depends on I:E ratio)[‡] |

[‡] If the inspiratory time is 0.5 s and the expiratory time is 1.0 s then the I:E ratio would be 1:2 and the expression $I+(E/I) = 1 + 2/1 = 3$

[*] Coaxial system 1.   Reservoir bag on inspiratory side
   2.   Reservoir bag on expiratory side with expiratory valve
   3.   Open ended reservoir bag on expiratory side

[†] Ventilation with the Mapleson A circuit can be achieved by
   1. Partially closing the expiratory relief valve and allowing a leak during the inspiratory phase
   2. Completely closing the expiratory relief valve during the inspiratory phase—Carden/M.I.E. ventilator
   3. By using an injector positioned between the catheter mount and the breathing system—this entrains gas from the system during inspiration and thus the flow pattern is similar to that during spontaneous ventilation

Fresh gas delivery tubing may be of narrow bore, hence high resistance, but all breathing hose has to be of low resistance. In the Bain system the delivery hose is the central tube, in the Lack it is the outer circumferential space, the inner tube being the expiratory hose. Because of the flow characteristics of the Mapleson A type both inner and outer conduits of the Lack system must be of low resistance.

### 2.  With carbon dioxide absorption
Soda lime is used to remove carbon dioxide from the breathing system.

It consists of    90%   $Ca(OH)_2$
   5%   NaOH
   1%   KOH

Silicates are added to prevent powdering and there is some moisture present to encourage the chemical reaction.

$$CO_2 + 2NaOH \rightarrow H_2O + Na_2CO_3 + heat$$

$$Na_2CO_3 + Ca(OH)_2 \rightarrow 2NaOH + CaCO_3 + heat$$

4–8 mesh granules are used to minimise the resistance to breathing but at the same time providing plenty of surface area for absorption. Resistance should be less than 2–3 cmH$_2$O at normal tidal flows.

a) *To and fro system* (Water's)

| Advantage | compactness |
|---|---|
| Disadvantages | 1. Absorber near patient's head—unwieldy |
| | 2. Apparatus dead space is high (200 ml) |
| | 3. Channelling of gas through soda-lime due to horizontal position of canister |
| | 4. Danger of inhalation of dust |
| | 5. If $V_T$ < volume of soda lime canister the proximal granules become exhausted and the dead space rises |

b) *Circle systems*

These systems may be semi-closed or, more rarely, totally closed. It is usual for the vaporiser to be outside the circle in the semi-closed system; however, there is renewed interest in the direct injection of the volatile anaesthetic liquid into the circuit.

The lower the fresh gas flow the more likely are large variations from the delivered gas concentrations in the circle; therefore monitoring of the oxygen concentration in the inspired gas is essential. These variations occur because of different rates of uptake of gases in the mixture.

When the circle system is used for paediatric anaesthesia the gas can be forced around the circuit by a fan—a Revell circulator to ensure removal of carbon dioxide.

When using a totally closed system, none of the inhalational anaesthetic is wasted. It is therefore possible to predict very accurately the amount of volatile agent required per unit time.

The advantages of the low flow circle system are economy, humidification and stability of inhaled gas concentration once the initial equilibration phase is over. A disadvantage is that intubation is mandatory when using very low flows—to ensure a good seal. The carbon dioxide absorber is positioned vertically to reduce the likelihood of channelling of gas through the granules.

The pressure at which the relief valve operates to protect the rotameters and vaporisers (35 kPa), is too high to protect the patient's airway and therefore another valve should be incorporated in the breathing system to protect the patient in the event of obstruction to the gas outflow. This pressure limiting valve should be set at 4–6 kPa (40–60 $cmH_2O$).

## SCAVENGING

There is still debate about the long term effects of low concentrations of anaesthetic agents in the environment but it is considered desirable to exhaust all waste anaesthetic gases away from working areas.

There is some evidence that the effects of chronic exposure to anaesthetic agents are:
1. Obstetric
   Increased risk of miscarriage
   Premature deliveries
2. Headache and fatigue
3. Increased incidence of malignancy in lymphoid tissue

As a gas leaves the breathing system it is ducted away, either passively or actively. Passive systems have the advantage of simplicity but exhausting the gases to the outside of buildings is not without difficulty e.g. wind direction and nesting birds. Active systems are complex and require high flows and negative pressures which are only slightly below those in the breathing system. Excessive negative pressure may empty the reservoir bag and therefore low flow circuits become impracticable. The requirement for high-flow scavenging may be reduced by using a reservoir bag in the system—to take the dumped gas during expiration and thereby even out the fluctuations during the respiratory cycle.

Obstruction of the scavenging tubing prevents the exhaust of the waste gases which may lead to an excessively high pressure in the airway. This can be prevented by having a safety discharge valve in the scavenging system close to the patient, opening at 0.5–1.0 kPa (5–10 $cmH_2O$).

The removal of volatile agents by passing exhausted gas through activated charcoal is an alternative method. Nitrous oxide is not removed, and trichloroethylene is not removed very efficiently. The life of a single charcoal canister depends on the concentration of vapours passing through it, and is generally about 3–6 h. Some canisters can be recycled by passing them through an autoclave—this removes the vapour, reactivating the charcoal and exhausting the wasted gas. Exhaustion of charcoal canister can be determined by weight.

The vacuum pumps used to extract the gases have to be resistent to the effects of the vapours—trichloroethylene, for example, is a potent degreasing agent and used as such in industry.

## VENTILATORS

Ventilators are machines designed to deliver a mixture of gases to patients in such a way that oxygen uptake and carbon dioxide elimination are maintained through the lungs. There is no simple classification, due to design variations. Hunter (1961), Mushin et al (1969) and Grogono (1972) have each attempted their own taxonomy.

Hunter's classification was based on whether tidal volume or airway pressure was preset, Mushin's depended on the constancy of the flow or pressure and the method of cycling, and Grogono's was based on whether the machine's function was independent of the patient's changing respiratory state.

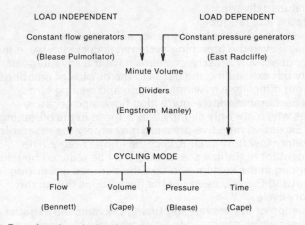

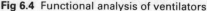

**Fig 6.4** Functional analysis of ventilators

Constant flow machines produce linear changes in airway pressure, i.e. the lung volume rises linearly because of the constant flow and therefore the airway pressure will also rise linearly, assuming constant compliance. These machines cannot compensate for leaks.

Constant pressure machines produce exponential changes in airway pressure; compensation for leaks occurs within limits.

Minute volume dividers, at a given rate, will produce a given airway pressure. This is because rate determines tidal volume, and tidal volume/compliance equals pressure.

Ideally a ventilator should be able to maintain the minute ventilation of a patient whether there is an obstruction or a leak. When a change in one ventilatory parameter is made, the others should remain constant, e.g. a change in tidal volume should not produce a change in respiratory rate. They should also be reliable, stable, flexible and simple to operate. Monitoring and warning devices should be available and the respiratory circuits should be capable of being removed for sterilising. Compression of gases within the machine and respiratory hoses can account for 20% of the tidal volume.

Ventilators for paediatric use should have a range of tidal volume from 10–150 ml, with rates from 30–120 min$^{-1}$.

There are specific machines for use with neonates on special care baby units; however, adult machines can be adapted to manage the larger child, as follows:

1. A resistance may be inserted in parallel to the child. Some gas passes to the child and some through the resistance. This type of system acts like a pressure generator.
2. A compliance, e.g. a distensible bag, may be inserted in parallel. The disadvantage of this is that if the child's compliance falls then a greater volume will pass into the bag and the child's tidal volume will fall.
3. A bag or bellows in a bottle is a better arrangement—the fresh gas flow is completely separate from the adult respiratory circuit and determines the minute ventilation. The adult ventilator simply squeezes the bag or bellows within the bottle.

Trigger, intermittent mandatory ventilation (IMV) and mandatory minute ventilation (MMV) are three methods of weaning patients from ventilators.

A trigger is effective only if the response time of the ventilator to the patient's inspiratory effort is short enough to deliver the set tidal volume during the inspiratory effort, and not during the expiratory phase that follows. The pressure required to trigger the ventilator can be increased as the patient's respiratory ability improves.

IMV is a technique during which the mechanical tidal volume and frequency of ventilation are preset, the patient being free to breathe spontaneously between these mandatory inflations. However the patient may have difficulty in synchronising with the ventilator if the controlled breaths are too infrequent.

MMV is a similar system but in this arrangement the total minute ventilation is determined by the fresh gas flow. Gas which the patient does not breathe spontaneously is diverted to a minute volume divider and is used to ventilate the patient mechanically. This system ensures a fixed minute volume, thereby reducing the likelihood of carbon dioxide retention or hypoxia.

Some clinicians consider artificial means of weaning as inappropriate and consider that the patient will breathe spontaneously when ready to do so.

## HUMIDIFIERS

The water content of inspired gas should approach 44 mg.l$^{-1}$ (100% relative humidity at 37°C).

1. Rebreathing systems—To and Fro      40–100% saturation
                         Circle      40– 60% saturation
2. Swedish 'Nose'—heat and moisture      40– 90% saturation
   exchanger
3. Water bath humidifiers      100% saturation
4. Mechanical nebulisation      100% saturation
5. Ultrasonic nebulisation      >150% saturation possible

3. (continued) When bubbling gas through, or over, heated water it becomes 100% saturated at that temperature. As the gas passes towards the patient it will cool and water will condense out. However, 100% humidity is still maintained, though the quantity of water is reduced. The temperature of the gas entering the patient should be monitored.

4. (continued). Baffles are used to break up droplets, and 80% of those droplets inhaled are between 2 and 4 $\mu$m. These are deposited mainly in the upper airways.

5. (Continued). A crystal vibrating at a frequency of about 3 MHz nebulises droplets of water. 70% of these particles will be between 0.8 and 1 $\mu$m. Overhydration is possible, increases in airway resistance has been described and cross infection by contamination of the droplet aerosol has been demonstrated.

Water vapour is the ideal mode of humidification (no droplets = no cross-infection), but if droplet aerosols are used then the optimal size of droplet is about 3–8 $\mu$m.

## FILTERS

### Gas

Filters are used in high-pressure gas lines to protect the ventilator control circuits against dirt, particularly if they are under fluidic control; other filters are found on some ventilator air entrainment inlets.

The use of bacterial gas filters within the breathing circuit is now common. Their use reduces, or avoids, the necessity for ventilator sterilisation and protects the patient from airborne cross-infection. Water logging of the filter increases airway resistance and facilitates the passage of bacteria through the filter. This problem has now been overcome by siliconising the filter element, a water-repellent material. Those filters that are not disposable are autoclaved daily.

## Liquid

Filters may be used to prevent the entry into the circulation of a variety of small particles found in intravenous infusions and drugs; metal, glass, fibres, moulds and even diatoms and insects. The pore size used is 2 $\mu$m and thus acts also as a bacterial filter. Flow rates through the filter are low and some debris can be dislodged from the filter itself. Filters are not used routinely for intravenous infusions but are generally used for the administration of epidural local anaesthetics.

## Blood filters

Aggregates in blood can be very large—up to 160 $\mu$m. The filtration of particles down to 40 $\mu$m in size removes these aggregates and allows the normal cellular material to pass through. Some filters have a pore size of 20 $\mu$m.

There are two types; screen filters and depth filters—the former are of large surface area (by multiple folds in a single layer of screen) but suffer the disadvantage of pore occlusion; however at high flows aggregates are not forced through. The depth filters filter aggregates by adsorbing them on tangled meshes of fibres; they tend to clog less but at high flow particles may be dislodged.

The case for their use is unproven, except possibly for transfusions in excess of 4 units of blood.

## ENDOTRACHEAL TUBES

There are many designs of endotracheal tubes. The general considerations determining their construction follow:
MATERIAL
Red Rubber —not normally disposable
—relatively irritant, not ideal for prolonged intubation
—firm/curvature predetermined
Plastic (PVC)—disposable
—non irritant
(implantation tested)
—moulds to body contours at 37°C

## Cuffs

Red rubber cuffs are firm and rounded so that a seal between endotracheal tube and trachea exists only over a small area. The mucosa is likely to be damaged, not only because of the chemical irritants but also because of compression, hence anoxia, of the mucosa.

PVC tubes have cuffs of varying shapes. The shape of the cuff can be more cylindrical thus increasing the area of seal, and thus reducing the required pressure within the cuff.

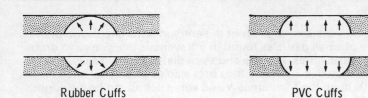

Rubber Cuffs                    PVC Cuffs

**Fig. 6.5** Endotracheal cuff characteristics

The seal between tracheal mucosa and endotracheal tube is required to prevent the escape of gas (during IPPV) and also prevent the aspiration of saliva or gastric contents into the tracheobronchial tree.

With low pressure cuffs the factors that determine whether a leak will occur are:
1. the pressure in the cuff
2. the length of the cuff
3. the cohesive force between the cuff material and the mucosa, dependent on surface tension
4. the duration of the inspiratory phase (the elevated pressure); the longer the pressure is applied then more of the cuff will be 'stripped' away from the mucosa and the greater the likelihood of a leak

Leakage of fluid from above past the cuff into the trachea depends on the head of pressure involved, and also possible movement of fluid between the cuff and the tracheal wall in capillary-like channels.

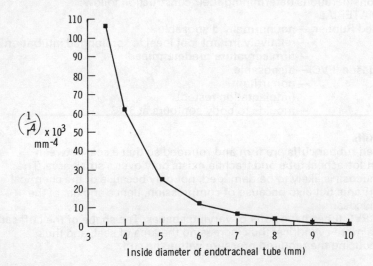

$$\left(\frac{1}{r^4}\right) \times 10^3 \text{ mm}^{-4}$$

Inside diameter of endotracheal tube (mm)

**Fig 6.6** Resistance to flow versus internal diameter of endotracheal tubes

**Size**

The outside diameter of the tube determines the smallest lumen into which it can be passed; the inside diameter together with the length estimates to air-flow resistance and hence to the work of breathing. Resistance is measured as the pressure drop in cm of water along the tube at a given flow of gas, standard measurements are made at a flow of 40 l.min$^{-1}$.

It can be seen from Figure 6.6 that, for tubes with an inside diameter of greater than 7 mm, small increases in the inside diameter do not confer much advantage in terms of flow, as $r^4$, although large, increases at a declining rate.

Age/4 + 4.5 is the accepted formula for determining the size of the endotracheal tube, in mm, for a child.

The length of the tube is determined by

Age/2 + 12 cm (oral)

Age/2 + 15 cm (nasal)

For infants the largest endotracheal tube should be passed that will fit the cricoid ring, the narrowest part of the child's airway. In tubes of small diameter, as required for infants, for a small difference in diameter there is a relatively marked change in the resistance to air flow during breathing.

Below the age of 10 it is often considered unnecessary to use cuffed tubes; this reduces subglottic damage and enables the use of a tube of larger diameter. The tube should not be a tight fit.

Gas flow in endotracheal tubes with a smooth and regular inner surface is laminar at flow rates less than the critical velocity. A small tube which is contaminated with debris will induce turbulent flow. Angled connectors also produce turbulence.

There are many different tubes; the common paediatric ones are:
1. Magill flexometallic
2. Cole
3. Plain Magill
4. Portex
5. Oxford
6. Jackson Rees

There are many specialised tubes used in adults.
1. Red rubber reinforced, styllete introducer required
2. PVC reinforced
3. Pollard and Coplans—for laryngeal microsurgery
4. Montando—for laryngectomy
5. Oxford
6. Carden—for intra-tracheal jet ventilation
7. Endobronchial/double lumen tubes (see Table 6.1)
8. Oesophageal obturator—for emergency resuscitation

**Table 4** Methods available for producing bronchial blockade
Right lung to be collapsed

| Single lumen tube | Double lumen tube | Bronchus blocker |
|---|---|---|
| Machray modification[*1] Magill endobronchial tube in left main bronchus | Carlen's tube | Vernon Thompson[$3] blocker right main bronchus + endotracheal tube |
| Magill endobronchial[*1] tube in the left main bronchus | Bryce-Smith/Salt[†2] tube into right main bronchus | Magill bronchus[$3] occluder + endotracheal tube |
| MacIntosh-Leatherdale left endobroncheal tube | Bryce-Smith tube into left main bronchus | |
| Brompton-Pallister left sided with one cuff on tracheal tube and two on bronchial | Left sided Robertshaw tube | |
| | White right-sided[†2] (carinal hook) | |

Left lung to be collapsed

| Single lumen tube | Double lumen tube | Bronchus blocker |
|---|---|---|
| | Carlen's tube[†2] | Vernon Thompson[$3] blocker left main bronchus + endotracheal tube |
| Magill right tube[*1] with wire coil | Bryce-Smith/Salt tube into right main bronchus allows ventilation of right upper lobe | Magill bronchus occluder + endotracheal tube |
| MacIntosh/Leatherdale left bronchus blocker & combined endotracheal tube | Bryce-Smith tube[†2] into left main bronchus | |
| Gordon/Green right sided tube (allows ventilation right upper lobe) | Right sided Robertshaw tube | |
| | White right-sided permits ventilation right upper lobe (carinal hook) | |

[1*] must be introduced over bronchoscope
[2†] although can be used for this purpose-best avoided for pneumonectomy
[$3] must be introduced through bronchoscope

For right upper lobectomy:
1. Magill bronchus occluder plus endotracheal tube
2. Vellacott right sided tube ⎫   allowing ventilation of right
                              ⎬   middle and
3. Green right-sided tube    ⎭   lower lobes and left lung

Reproduced, with permission of the authors and publishers, from Thornton J A, Levy C J Techniques of Anaesthesia. Chapman & Hall, London.

## LARYNGOSCOPES

There are many designs for use depending on requirement:

### 1. Neonatal—straight blade
The epiglottis is relatively large and floppy; a straight blade is necessary to flatten and hold the epiglottis forward to allow the cords to be visualised.

### 2. Infant—straight or curved blade
The tongue of the infant is large in relation to the buccal cavity and blade design is aimed at keeping it out of the way. Blades which are almost tubular are used in infants with tissue flaps associated with palatal defects. The most commonly used paediatric laryngoscopes are the Anderson–Magill and the Robertshaw.

### 3. Adult—straight or curved blade
The primary aim is deflection of the tongue from the line of vision of the vocal cords however a variety of other problems have been overcome.
a) A laryngoscope with an obtuse angle between the handle and the blade—to facilitate insertion into the mouths of patients with difficult access, i.e. in an iron lung, in severe fixed flexion or in a halo splint for stabilisation of the cervical spine
b) A 'left handed blade'—for use in patients where the right side of the mouth is invaded by tumour, or access otherwise compromised
c) The addition of a prism to the blade allows the vocal cords to be visualised when they are not in direct line of sight

### 4. Fibreoptic laryngoscope
A thin flexible fibreoptic device that will pass through a size 8.0 mm endotracheal tube. It may be helpful if intubation is difficult, and by its use the tube can be directed in the appropriate direction.

# Index

٧٧٢
٠.٩